HANNAH'S PRAYER

HANNAH'S PRAYER

(A 31-day Devotional for Supernatural Conception)

TOMI ADISA

DAY 8
GOD HAS REMEMBERED ME

DAY 9
STRENGTHEN ME, O GOD

DAY 10
I CAN SEE, AND I WILL CARRY MY CHILDREN

DAY 11
I CANCEL EVERY NEGATIVE DREAM

DAY 12
I UPROOT WHATEVER GOD HAS NOT PLANTED IN MY BODY AND MY HUSBAND'S BODY

DAY 13
I BREAK EVERY NEGATIVE GENERATIONAL PATTERN

DAY 14
LORD, HONOUR YOUR WORD IN MY LIFE

DAY 15
I AM ANOINTED TO BE FRUITFUL

DAY 16
I REBUKE THE SPIRIT OF DEATH

DAY 17

MY BODY IS QUICKENED

DAY 18

I CANCEL EVERY NEGATIVE UTTERANCE

DAY 19

I ACTIVATE EVERY PROPHECY SPOKEN INTO MY LIFE

DAY 20

THE LORD HEARS ME, AND HE WILL ANSWER ME

DAY 21

SUPERNATURAL FINANCIAL PROSPERITY

DAY 22

EVERY HIDDEN HEALTH PROBLEM IS EXPOSED

DAY 23

I WILL NOT MISCARRY MY BABIES

DAY 24

I WILL NOT GIVE UP ON GOD

PREFACE

One night in April 2023, as I lay on my bed, I heard the words 'Hannah's Offering' in my spirit. Immediately, without much thinking, I responded as though to correct the thought and said ' Hannah's Prayers', but the Lord repeated Himself and said 'Hannah's Offering.'

Then the Lord explained that Hannah's Prayers were not just prayers but also an offering. She brought her pain, brokenness and faith amidst tears to God. Indeed, our prayers rise to God as incense.

God knows that some days will be tough, and He permits us to bring our pain just as we bring our joy, our fears just as we bring our faith, and our sorrows just as we bring our peace. God accepts our prayers if we pray in faith. The prayer of faith can be filled with tears. Even Jesus wept as He prayed (Luke 22:44), and God heard and strengthened Him.
Prayer must be vulnerable so that God can comfort you.

Like Hannah, when we choose to pray amid great pain, our prayers rise to God as incense. It is a great sacrifice to pray when we feel pain, and God does not take it lightly. God knows that the flesh is tempted to find comfort in other things when in pain. Therefore, God greatly respects the prayers sown in tears and agony of heart. God had great respect for the offerings of Hannah; she brought everything she had even though she had almost nothing. This is how the title of this book came to be.
God does not take lightly the offerings and prayers of Hannah.

I have stood with friends, sisters and church members trusting God for a child, and I know it's a tough walk. It is no small thing to wait for a child; it can be hard. I think it is the hardest wait.

I have, sometimes, felt like charging God to court because of the pain I feel for those who wait. I felt great pain listening to the despair of women who have had miscarriages.

I have also seen God too many times to count, turning an impossible situation around. God has done many supernatural conceptions, and I have honestly lost count.
Restored ovulation, menstrual flow regulated, fibroid disappeared, and supernatural conceptions of all kinds against negative medical reports! **God is faithful.**

I have seen raw miracles that left me dumbfounded! I have seen and heard many! God cannot be underestimated.

No wonder the Bible says our light affliction cannot be compared to the glory ahead of us (2 Corinthians 4:17). This is why the prayers in this devotional are not religious; they are heartfelt.

I have written this book by the inspiration of God to families in God's Waiting Room, especially the women. I write as your sister - One who shares your pain and believes with you. I write to hold your hands and encourage you to have faith.

I write as a Warrior who has fought many battles and seen God's mighty hand too many times to doubt Him. I know GOD CAN BE TRUSTED.

I write as a Shepherd; one saddled with the responsibility of guiding God's people - a responsibility I take very seriously. I hope this book helps your heart and gives you the strength to believe.
If we have faith, we will see miracles.

I am sending you a big hug. I ask that you read every page like a letter from God because God is mindful of you. Your miracle is here, and you will testify in Jesus' name.

Send your testimony to tomiadisaministries@gmail.com

You are a joyful mother of many beautiful children in Jesus' name.
Amen

INTRODUCTION

Waiting is a part of life's cycle. No one, great or small, can escape waiting. Waiting is a privilege reserved for the Living; the dead can no longer wait. Waiting is a part of life's cycle.

The waiting room of life, especially for the promise of a child, can be challenging, lonely and painful. It is the joy and desire of every woman to carry her child—no woman dreams of waiting to conceive. Waiting is not easy, but it becomes bearable and profitable with the right perspective.

The right perspective gives us the right attitude. We must see waiting as a phase and not a death sentence. What you see is what you become; I encourage you to see well.

Everyone has waited, and everyone will wait. How, when, for how long and for what; nobody knows. One may be waiting for a life partner while another waits for a prodigal son to return; one can be waiting to be healed, while another waits for the fruit of the womb, and the list goes on.

No anointing or favour can exclude a man from waiting.

Waiting is how faith is built.

Every waiting mother in the Bible has a unique story to tell. From desperate Sarah, who succumbed to the cultural pressure of giving her maid to her husband, to fair Rachel, who put her husband in the position only God occupies, each of these women had to go through

God's waiting room to birth the child of His dreams, not theirs.

They had to learn to submit their desires, ambitions, expectations and shame on the altar and wait on God to do as He pleased. These women were some of the first partakers of the resurrection of the dead. They sowed their wombs and allowed God to use them for His pleasure. Paul described this mystery to the Corinthian church in this fashion.

And when it dies, God gives it a new form, a body to fulfil his purpose, and he sees to it that each seed gets a new body of its own and becomes the plant he designed it to be. 1 Corinthians 15:38 TPT

Are you also in the waiting room? Are you looking to Jesus to fulfil His promises concerning your miracle babies? They might be physical or spiritual babies because, in one way or the other, every woman is a waiter. You are in a good place because God is about to give your womb a new form, and your waiting is a preparation ground to birth His good pleasure.

You, too, will soon become a partaker of the resurrection of the dead because Jesus is the resurrection and life (John 11:25).

God's promises answer to His principles, and when you know how to work the principles that guide the waiting room, you will enjoy the fulfilment of God's promises. This book, Hannah's Prayers, is a 31-day devotional, and it will guide you on how to honour the Lord in your waiting season. Who we become is far more important than what we have. This devotional will also provide comfort, encouragement and help you articulate your needs in prayer.

As you pray with this devotional, you will find the faith to believe for the impossible and receive the courage to wait on God's Word and the strength to conceive and birth your seed, as Sarah did. You will learn practical steps from Hannah's life and the Scriptures to follow as you wait on the Lord and receive wisdom to maximize and steward your waiting process. You will know the loopholes to block and the windows to open to allow the fresh release of God's grace to permeate your heart and invigorate your soul as you wait.

And more importantly, you will know how to cooperate with God to hasten His Word to perform it.

Beloved, you are not the only one waiting; God is waiting too. He is waiting for you to get the divine gist and yield to Him as Hannah did. He is waiting to use your womb for His glory. Don't keep Him waiting any longer. Surrender, and let Him write His story through you.

Through faith, Sarah (put your name) herself received strength to conceive seed, and was delivered of a child when she was past age, because she judged him faithful who had promised. Hebrews 11:11 KJV.

YOU ARE NOT GUILTY!

When things don't go as expected, it often makes the future look bleak and compels us to focus on the past because we seek answers. We look to what we know, have done and where we have been to check if we left something undone or badly done.

Many women in the waiting room of God who have done abortion at one time or the other feel deeply guilty for their waiting. They feel responsible for the wait. Some think it's God punishing them for committing abortion while some believe the only child or children they were destined to have has been aborted and they may never have children of their own. This is not true.

Yes, abortion is a sin; it is murder in the eyes of God.

"Your eyes saw my unformed body; all the days ordained for me were written in your book before one of them came to be." - **Psalm 139:16**

Jeremiah 1:5 (KJV) *Before I formed thee in the belly I knew thee; and before thou camest forth out of the womb I sanctified thee, and I ordained thee a prophet unto the nations.*

From the time a child is formed in the womb, God sees a person and when that person is killed, God sees murder. If you are single and reading this book, I encourage you to live responsibly. There is no excuse for abortion unless medically advised because the life of a mother or child is threatened. If abortion is the only option to save your life LITERALLY, it is medically advised, with the support of your spouse, you can make an informed decision that is void of lies and selfish motives.

HOWEVER, if you aborted your pregnancy in order to avoid the responsibility of raising a child against the will of God, the Same God is willing to forgive you. God is a God of Mercy. Abortion is a sin like every other sin. In God's eyes; sin is sin. The one who lies has sinned like the one who fornicated. God is more than willing to forgive us our sins if we repent and ask for forgiveness. God will not only forgive you; He will also heal you.

If you committed abortion and you repented of it; it happened in the time of ignorance. You were ignorant. If you knew what you knew now; you would have done better. Now that you know better and have asked for His forgiveness; YOU ARE FORGIVEN.

God is too compassionate to hold it against you. He forgives us our sins when we confess and repent from them.

Psalms 103:8-13 (KJV) The LORD is merciful and gracious, slow to anger, and plenteous in mercy.
He will not always chide: neither will he keep his anger forever.
He hath not dealt with us after our sins; nor rewarded us according

to our iniquities.

For as the heaven is high above the earth, so great is his mercy toward them that fear him.

As far as the east is from the west, so far hath he removed our transgressions from us.

Like as a father pitieth his children, so the LORD pitieth them that fear him.

Psalms 86:5 (KJV) *For thou, Lord, art good, and ready to forgive; and plenteous in mercy unto all them that call upon thee.*

GOD HAS FORGIVEN YOU! I know the feeling of guilt is real and you may even have nightmares filled with the details of the abortion. The enemy can use your emotions to manipulate you. He will speak lies into your mind and make it sound like your thoughts. He is a Mind Trickster. Don't let your mind trick you into feeling guilty. You are forgiven and you must insist on it. Look to the Word of God that guarantees our liberty.

Romans 8:1 (KJV) *There is therefore now no condemnation to them which are in Christ Jesus, who walk not after the flesh, but after the Spirit.*

You must believe it! Like all things we believe God for; you must grow your faith. You must declare your pardon and redemption until you believe it without a shadow of doubt.

You must insist on your liberty.

Yes, the miscarriage may have happened because of a wrong decision you took but God has forgiven you. You do not deserve to suffer for something you already lost. God is a God of Restoration.

Let Him carry you.

If God wanted to punish us for our sins; God has the record of all our imperfections, He will do much more than the challenge you have interpreted as punishment.

Sodom and Gomorrah did worse yet God was willing to forgive them if he found repentance. Repentance is a game changer. Repentance makes God your ally when He should be your enemy. Look at David; he took the wife of a man who was committed to serving him and killed the man. God exposed his sin and David repented immediately. He put on sackcloth and humbled himself before God. He lost the child from the adultery but after his repentance; God blessed him with another child who became the wisest man on earth.

Don't let the devil lie to you. You are free from your sins. The next time the devil accuses you; make sure you open your mouth and tell him you have been pardoned by Jesus and washed clean of your sins by the blood of Jesus. Don't keep quiet in the face of accusations.

Matthew 26:28 (KJV) *For this is my blood of the new testament, which is shed for many for the remission of sins.*

The blood of Jesus cleansed you and through that blood all your sins are remitted.
You no longer have your sins and they no longer belong to you.
They are CANCELLED! That is what remission means.

When you feel guilty; remember that the devil is lying to you through your feelings. He is a terrible and wicked liar. You must be aggressive in declaring the TRUTH!

My dearest sis, this is the warfare you must engage in. Don't let the devil steal your confidence, faith and joy!

You are waiting; you are not condemned. You are waiting; you are not being punished. You are waiting; you are not abandoned. You are waiting; you are ignored. You are waiting; you are not rejected.

You are precious in the eyes of God and loved with an everlasting love.

Jeremiah 31:3 (KJV) The LORD hath appeared of old unto me, saying, Yea, I have loved thee with an everlasting love: therefore with lovingkindness have I drawn thee.
Remember, God can never fight anything that has been redeemed by the blood of Jesus. He cannot fight His own blood.

You have been redeemed. You are loved. You are free from the past. Now, live free.

Therefore, if anyone is in Christ, the new creation has come: The old has gone, the new is here! **2 Corinthians 5:17**

Now, that you are free from guilt and fear, pray with this devotional and pray confidently.

DAY 1

THANKSGIVING

TEXT: PSALM 95:1-2

REFLECTION:

Why should you give thanks in everything, especially as you wait?
(1 Thessalonians 5:18).

*And whatsoever you do in Word or deed, do all in the name of
Jesus, giving thanks to God and the Father by Him. Colossians
3:17 KJV.*

Thanksgiving doesn't come naturally in the waiting room.
Complaining, comparison, murmuring, and arguing does.
The natural woman finds it easier to slide the downward path of
complaining, but you are not natural.
You are spiritual; as a spirit, you create divine atmospheres within

and around you by engaging kingdom principles.

Thanksgiving is a powerful kingdom principle that sets the stage for miracles. It shuts out negative voices and magnifies God's good nature. It redirects your heart to see what God has done in the past, what He can do, and how limitless and powerful He is.

When you thank God for your season, you invite Him to change them for your good and His glory. Regardless of the number of years you have waited, the negative reports you have received, the jeers, mockery and insults, choose to give God thanks because thanksgiving is not just God's will; it births God's perfect will.

Thanksgiving sets you above your circumstances. It not only honours and glorifies God; it also gives you joy—the joy you need to be strong in your waiting season.

Thanksgiving silences the enemy. If you don't praise God, you will find yourself murmuring, worrying, complaining and engaging in every wicked thing the enemy plants in your heart. Thanksgiving is how you take charge and enthrone God above all!

PRAYER

1. My soul magnifies You, Lord. I thank You for my process and Your promises.
   I thank You for Your unfailing love and grace. I am grateful because You have a track record of keeping Your Word.
   I put on the garment of thanksgiving, and never will I put it off again. Out of my mouth will proceed songs of praise and thanksgiving to my God. Amen.

2. Lord, I thank you for the gift of life and salvation. Every day, you watch over me and keep me safe. You have given your angels charge over me. You have given me life abundantly. I have the Zoe life; because of this, I am victorious.

3. Lord, I thank you for the grace to wait and not give up. You are my strength and sustenance. It is by your power that I am standing today. You are my pillar and covering.

4. Lord, I thank you for peace in my home. Thank you for my husband and the life you have given us together. Thank you, Jesus, because the love in my marriage will only grow stronger in this phase. Thank you for my husband, for strengthening him and helping him to believe in your Word. Thank you for victory over every attack of the enemy against my marriage.

5. Lord, with the whole of my heart, I thank you for giving me a sound mind. The enemy tried to take my mind but failed because You watch over me and don't sleep nor slumber.

6. Thank you for giving me the strength to face every day, especially those that mock me, situations that remind me, and very difficult days. Without you, I would have collapsed. You have been my Pillar and Core. Thank you for giving me the courage to overcome the mockery of the godless. I know my testimony will come.

7. Lord, I thank You because my life will always glorify You no matter what I face. I thank You for the privilege to serve Your will. I thank You for the gift of my children because I know You did not create me to be barren. I thank You for my womb will carry and birth many children. I am a joyful mother of children. Amen!

I BELIEVE GOD'S REPORT

TEXT: HEBREWS 12:1-2

REFLECTION

Whose report will you believe?

Faith, then, is birthed in a heart that responds to God's anointed utterance of the Anointed One. Romans 10:17 TPT

Waiting is hard! Let no one tell you waiting is easy. Waiting is hard, but it is not impossible. We have seen great heroes of faith in the Bible who hoped against hope. In our time, we have heard unbelievable testimonies of men and women who stood against doctor's reports to receive their babies or dead family members back to life.

There is no limit to what God can do if we dare to believe.

Science, Google, family, society and self-reports can keep you from receiving God's promises if you choose to listen to and believe them because your life will go in the direction of your word and beliefs. God's report is in His Word, and He will not allow any of His Word to fall to the ground without fulfilling what He has sent it to accomplish. (Isaiah 55:11).

You must choose to hold fast to God's Word, to believe His report about Himself and His report about you. God doesn't answer to what others have said about you, nor does he answer to what you have said about yourself. He responds to His Word, and rest assured that when you believe His Word, He will answer to you.

Faith comes by hearing God's Word. The more you expose yourself to God's Word, the surer you become about His promises. God has given you everything you need to build a defence of faith against negative reports. Stay in His Word until your heart becomes an impenetrable fortress against the devil's lies concerning your life.

As sure as the Lord lives, you are going to testify. You will share your testimony with me very soon. I already see how you will dance at your baby's christening ceremony. Can you see it?

When you believe the report of God, you begin to see differently. From today, you will believe again.

PRAYER

1. Lord, I believe in Your Word concerning all that concerns me. My womb, body, mind, heart, husband, (add other things) align with what You have said and are saying. I am fruitful, and I multiply. I bring forth after God's kind and defy all negative reports. I only believe the report of the Lord. Amen.

2. By the Word of God in Exodus 23:26, I will not be barren or cast my young. The last time I had a miscarriage is the last time I will ever miscarry my seed. My body and womb are empowered to conceive and carry to term in Jesus' name.

3. I believe the report of the Lord that says my body is the temple of the Lord. Therefore, no ailment, infirmity or sickness can stay in my body. My body is blessed because it is the dwelling place of Yahweh. (1 Corinthians 6:19-20).

4. I am not who men say I am. I am who God says I am. I am not the doctor's report. Your Word says I am fruitful (Genesis 9:7). I am a joyful mother whose children surround her table (Psalm 113:9). I am not barren. (Deuteronomy 7:14). I am blessed and highly favoured by God and men (Luke 1:28), and THAT'S WHO I AM!

5. I declare the report of the Lord concerning my body. It is anointed to carry babies and carry them till birth. My babies are healthy and strong, and they live. My womb is now opened to carry my babies. My husband's body is anointed to release living seeds. My husband's body suffers no limitation. My are empowered to conceive and carry to term in Jesus' name.

6. I declare the report of the Lord that light shines upon every darkness in my life. Whatever way the enemy has been afflicting me that is hidden from me, today, light shines upon it in Jesus' name. It is revealed in a dream. It is revealed to the doctors. I come against every ignorance contending with my Fruitfulness in Jesus' name.

7. This is the report of the Lord. I am fruitful, and I multiply. I am carrying my babies. God has looked upon me with favour and has opened my womb. I am a mother of a lovely baby boy, baby girl, twins, triplets, quadruplets etc. I conceive this year, I carry to term and deliver safely in Jesus' name. Amen!!!

DAY 3

I WILL NOT GIVE UP; I WAIT ON THE LORD

TEXT: PSALM 27:13-14

REFLECTION

Why must you keep holding on?

But those who wait upon God get fresh strength. They spread their wings and soar like eagles, they run and don't get tired, they walk and don't lag behind. Isaiah 40:31 MSG

Waiting is not easy on the flesh because it is designed to kill your carnal desires and selfish ambitions. Hannah discovered this truth the hard way. She had to wait until she shed the last skin of her self-driven desire for a child. Just as God dealt in love with Hannah, God loves you too much to allow you to birth something that doesn't look like His will.

And because of His love, He will teach you to wait correctly.

Your willpower, strength or abilities are insufficient to help you persevere in the waiting room. God has a curriculum He wants you to follow in this room, and only His grace is sufficient to help you through. Without Him, you will faint, give up and fail, but your strength is renewed in Him, and you soar like an eagle into the sunrise of His promises.

You are an eagle, beloved, and giving up is not part of your DNA. No matter how tough the waiting gets, God's strength in you is tougher and stronger. His grace is sufficient to help you keep holding on even when the night seems longer than usual. And whenever you feel like giving up, know it is time to lean more on the Lord. Don't be weary as you wait because, in due time, you will reap if you don't faint. (Galatians 6:9). You will carry your babies (physical and spiritual) soon.

On tough days, remember the Lord is close to the brokenhearted and wants to comfort you. (Psalms 34:18). God has also surrounded you with angels, men and women who can hold your hand, pray with you and comfort you.

May you find great encouragement on dark and lonely days, in Jesus' name.

PRAYER

1. Thank you, Lord, for sustaining me. I would have lost my mind, given up and completely turned away if you had not been on my side. The enemy would have consumed me. Lord, you are my pillar and my strength. Lord, I am so grateful for your Presence, love and peace.

2. Dear Jesus, my eyes are on You. I hope and wait on You with all my heart, regardless of how I feel. I will not be weary because I am an eagle, and fainting or giving up is not part of my DNA. I rest in Your love and promises and know I will never be ashamed. Amen.

3. Lord, I ask for strength this season –the strength to remain in your love, persevere, be at peace, forgive those who mock me, stay believing, and hold my peace in Jesus' name. Lord, by your strength, I will not faint in the days of adversity. My strength will not be small in Jesus' name. I will mount up with wings as the eagle in Jesus' name.

4. Lord, open my eyes to see the wonderful future you have for me. Lord, I need to see the glory set ahead of me. I know your thoughts towards me are always of peace and not of evil. (Jeremiah 29:11).

5. Let my eyes see a future filled with many children, grandchildren and great-grandchildren. Lord, as you showed Abraham the stars and renewed your promise to him, let my faith be strengthened as well.

6. Lord Jesus, I receive encouragement from you today in Jesus' name. Let everything that can encourage a man waiting on the Lord be released to me today in Jesus' name. I will not faint or be weary in Jesus' name. My encouragement has come.

7. Lord Jesus, you are the lifter of my head. I will not bow my head in shame in Jesus' name. I will remember your tender mercies and stay hopeful. I will hope against hope like Abraham. I will wake up every day believing that my miracle has come. I will not give my attention to those who hate and despise me in Jesus' name.

8. This is the report of the Lord. I am fruitful, and I multiply. I am carrying my babies. God has looked upon me with favour and has opened my womb. I am a mother of a lovely baby boy, baby girl, twins, triplets, quadruplets etc. I conceive this year, I carry to term and deliver safely in Jesus' name. Amen!!! With God, nothing is impossible. (Luke 1:37). Amen!

DAY 4

MY SPOUSE AND I REMAIN UNITED

TEXT: GENESIS 2:24

REFLECTION:

Why must you fight to keep the unity in your home?

But steadily, pouring yourselves out for each other in acts of love, alert at noticing differences and quick at mending fences. Ephesian 4:3 MSG

The waiting period is a sensitive and delicate phase that must be handled with care. The enemy's goal is not hidden. He comes to steal, kill and destroy, and he will prey on your ignorance and pride if you are not watchful.

If you were on a boat cruise alone with your spouse, and right in the middle of your adventure, you began arguing about something and exchanging words, what would you do if a storm suddenly arose? Will you continue your argument or find a way to escape the storm with your spouse? I am sure you will make the latter decision and probably postpone your disagreement until you land safely. Nobody in their right senses continues a petty fight in the face of a life-threatening storm.

I remember the story of a couple who trusted God for the fruit of the womb. They fought with each other every time the wife was ovulating. It was always one bad argument or the other during this period. Peace will return as soon as she starts her menstrual period. The wife, through revelation, began to pay attention to the timing of their disagreement. When she noticed the evil pattern, she decided to stop it.

The next time she and her husband had a bad argument during her ovulation, she ignored the fight and pressed her husband to be intimate with her.
That's how she became a mother. Sometimes, the miracle you seek is in your hands, but you can't see it. Disunity is a destructive agent.

Disunity is a life-threatening storm against any home; when you see it as the enemy that it is, you won't entertain it. Yes, you will disagree with your spouse on some things during your waiting season, but never allow it to escalate to the point of disunity. Don't break away from each other. Don't forget that you are together in this battle to birth God's will, and the devil wants to find a way to stop this from happening. If Joseph and Mary hadn't been on the same page, the birth of Jesus would have been truncated.

No matter what your spouse does or doesn't do, don't forget that he is not your enemy. Your enemy is satan, the deceiver and accuser of the brethren. When you disagree, guard your heart against the whispers of the devil. Don't invite him into the sharpening process and learning curves you are going through with your spouse. Firmly put him in his place – forever outside your home. When the enemy rears his ugly head to come into your home through division, crush his head with your prayers and humility. Do whatever it takes to be at peace with your husband. Peace is not the same as silence. Peace is choosing to be a team first before confronting any matter.

Unity is a system of advantage. Don't allow the devil to render you helpless. Your unity will hasten God's promises and make God trust your home with His will.

PRAYER

1. Lord, thank you for keeping my united despite our differences and preferences. Thank you for protecting us from the enemy. Thank you for giving us one mind, one voice and one love. Thank you, Jesus, for binding us together with your love.

2. As the gatekeeper of my home, I guard my gates against the dart of disunity. I agree with my spouse and never see him as my enemy. My husband will never see me as his enemy. We are united even in this waiting season, in Jesus' name. The unity of my home is kept and preserved in Jesus' name.

3. Together, we birth God's purposes on the earth, and God's Will prosper in our hands. My home is united, and I quickly mend broken fences in Jesus' name. Amen. My receive a humble heart to forgive quickly and remain united in Jesus' name.

4. In the name of Jesus, I silence every voice speaking against the unity of my home. I curse every desire to see my husband, and I separated. I decree that no weapon formed against my home will prosper in Jesus' name. (Isaiah 54:17). No man or woman will come between my in Jesus' name. Everyone waiting for the destruction of my home will be disappointed in Jesus' name.

5. I uproot anything God has not planted in my home in Jesus' name. Every seed of contention, fear, regret, malice, unforgiveness, misunderstanding etc, waiting to manifest later in my home is forever destroyed in Jesus' name.

6. My home will continue to flourish. This waiting season is a honeymoon season for my . We will fall deeper in love with each other. We will protect each other. We will pray for each other, honour and encourage each other. I am my husband's best friend, just as he is my best friend.

7. This is the report of the Lord. I am fruitful, and I multiply. I am carrying my babies. God has looked upon me with favour and has opened my womb. I am a mother of a lovely baby boy, baby girl, twins, triplets, quadruplets etc. I conceive this year, I carry to term and deliver safely in Jesus' name. Amen!!! My husband will carry our babies in Jesus' name. Amen!

DAY 5

I AM FRUITFUL
TEXT: GENESIS 1:26-28

REFLECTION:

What can stop you from bearing fruits when God calls you fruitful?

And I will make you exceeding fruitful, and I will make nations of thee, and kings shall come out of thee. Genesis 17:6 KJV

When God created the earth, He wrote fruitfulness as one of the codes to guide its operations. And when man was created, God commanded him to prosper, reproduce, fill the earth and take charge! Fruitfulness is one of your modus operandi as God's creation. In fact, it is a command you must obey. You cannot but bear fruits.

You are designed to bear fruit.

You are anointed to bear fruit. You are equipped to bear fruit, and you are ready to bear fruit. Fruitfulness is your God-ordained destiny! The birth of your children is not subject to other people's decisions, negative generational patterns, medical conclusions or your opinions. It is God's call and commandment for you to be fruitful.

God expects and demands that we be fruitful. Jesus showed us God's reaction to fruitlessness when he cursed the fig tree. We also see in John 15 that God pays attention to fruitfulness. God is invested in your fruitfulness.

Speak to your body today. Tell your womb what God has commanded it to be and do. You are a speaking spirit, and as long as your words align with God's will, you will have whatsoever you say. Apart from God, who knows no impossibility, there is nothing impossible to the woman that believes. (Mark 9:23).

Remember Mary's words and keep proclaiming what God has said. She said, *'And blessed is she that believed: for there shall be a performance of those things which were told her of the Lord.'* Luke 1:45 KJV. Keep telling every organ in your body to obey God's command because there shall be a performance of your fruitfulness.

PRAYER

1. Father in Heaven, I praise You because You have chosen, anointed and equipped me to be Fruitful. Without your Word, I would be barren, but because of what you said and what is written, I know for sure that I will bear fruits in my body. I will carry my babies, birth them and nurse them at my breast in Jesus' name.

2. I decree that everything in my body and my husband's body align with the Word of the Lord in Genesis 17:16. My are exceedingly fruitful in Jesus' name. A new day has come -the day of our Fruitfulness- in Jesus' name.

3. I am fruitful, exceeding fruitful, and nations proceed from my loins. I birth kings and queens that represent God's Kingdom on earth. All my organs obey God's command to be fruitful and multiply. Thank You, Jesus, for the performance of Your promises. It happens to me as You have commanded. Amen.

4. I hear the sound of my children laughing, playing, running and dancing in my home because I am fruitful. I see (insert the names of your children) in my home. They surround my table. I am a joyful mother of children in Jesus' name.

5. Everything standing in the way of my fruitfulness is uprooted in Jesus' name. It does not matter the weapon the enemy fashioned against me; I nullify them in Jesus' name. Every stronghold of barrenness is destroyed in my life in Jesus' name. I am fruitful in Jesus' name.

6. The blessing of the Lord is upon my life and has made me fruitful. Everything in my body and my husband's body is

empowered to conceive in Jesus' name. Every cell, tissue, organ, system, blood, water and bone is anointed to make me fruitful.

7. This is the report of the Lord. I am fruitful, and I multiply. I am carrying my babies. God has looked upon me with favour and has opened my womb. I am a mother of a lovely baby boy, baby girl, twins, triplets, quadruplets etc. I conceive this year, I carry to term and deliver safely in Jesus' name. Amen!!! My husband will carry our babies in Jesus' name. Amen!

DAY 6

I CANCEL EVERY DOCTOR'S REPORT

TEXT: EXODUS 14:14

REFLECTION:

Is that medical report more believable than God's Word?

Nobody speaks and it comes to pass unless the Lord has decreed it.
Lamentations 3:37 Tree of Life version.

When a monarch makes a decree, nobody, no matter how highly placed, can refute it. When Queen Vashti misbehaved, and the king decreed her banishment from the palace, his commandment was written among the laws of the Persians and Medians that could never be altered. If an earthly kingdom set things in place to ensure that the decrees of their mortal kings went unchallenged, how much more the decrees of the Monarch of Zion?!

Has a doctor's report written you off? Have you received laboratory tests that have tested your faith? Don't despair; no decree or report will stand when God is not the author. Let me remind you of two of God's decrees concerning you:

God's Word: Dig ditches all over this valley. Here's what will happen – you won't hear the wind, you won't see the rain, but this valley is going to fill up with water, and your army and your animals will drink their fill. 2 Kings 3:17 MSG.

Shout, and celebrate, Daughter of Zion! I'm on my way. I am moving into your neighbourhood! God's decree. Zechariah 2:10 MSG

Let God have the only laugh in your life. His laughter is in your favour and against every report that dares to speak against your fruitfulness. No written or unwritten doctor's report can stand when the Monarch of Zion has decreed in your favour. Absolutely none!

We have seen God do the impossible before. Mary conceived without the aid of a sperm. Low sperm count cannot stop you from carrying your babies if Mary could conceive with no sperm count because God counts more than anything else.

Sarah, in her old age, after she had long passed menopause and was even at 'menostop', conceived and gave birth to a bouncing baby boy. You will laugh just as Sarah laughed.

We have heard many testimonies of women without wombs carrying their babies. We have also heard of women whose doctors said their babies had no heartbeat receiving their dead back to life. Some women whose doctors said they were carrying a fibroid received their miracle child when God turned the fibroid into a fine boy. God is not limited by man, and that's why He is the only Living God.

PRAYER

1. With joy, I will sing your praises. You are God, and there is no place for any argument about your sovereignty. You can make a way where there was no way in Your sovereignty. You can raise the dead that has been dead for four days. You can open any door. You can open the eyes of the blind. You are the Almighty God. You are the Most High God. All reports are subject to you, and they bow at your feet in Jesus' name.

2. From today, I agree with your report only. My confession and meditation align with your report only. I will only think of the things that are possible, pure, true, beautiful, divine and lovely. (Philippians 4:8).

3. As your beloved daughter, Monarch of Zion, I only give ear to Your decrees concerning my life. You have decreed my health, joy, peace, fruitfulness and fullness, and I believe You alone. I lay every doctor's report at Your feet and see You turning them around for my good. Every negative report becomes a positive testimony to the glory of God. Amen.

4. In the name of Jesus, I cancel every negative report about my life. I silence the voice of evil reports and satanic declarations concerning my life in Jesus' name. Who has spoken when God has not decreed it?! I will not fear reports that don't align with the Word of God. My heart will firmly trust in Jesus. The doctors have spoken, but God has the Final Say.

The verdict is with my God, not man, and I believe in God with all my heart.

5. I will stand firm on the promises of God. I will not look at the mountain. I will look to the God who can make mountains plain. I will fix my gaze on Jesus and will not be ashamed.

6. I conceive this year, I carry to term and deliver safely in Jesus' name. Amen!!! I am returning with a new report, which will testify to my supernatural conception in Jesus' name.

7. This is the report of the Lord. I am fruitful, and I multiply. I am carrying my babies. God has looked upon me with favour and has opened my womb. I am a mother of a lovely baby boy, baby girl, twins, triplets, quadruplets etc. I conceive this year, I carry to term and deliver safely in Jesus' name. Amen!!! My husband will carry our babies in Jesus' name. Amen!

MY WOMB IS OPEN

TEXT: GENESIS 25:24

REFLECTION:

Who (or what) can shut what God has opened?

Shall I bring to birth, and not cause to bring forth? Saith the Lord:
shall I cause to bring forth, and shut the womb? Saith thy God?
Isaiah 66:9

No one or thing can close your womb when God calls you fruitful. Perhaps you don't even have a womb; that is a very small thing for God to do. God is the One who opens a door no man can shut, and He shuts a door no man can open.

Have you ever tried opening a door, and it didn't budge, only to discover that you didn't correctly set the key in the keyhole?

Whenever God sees alignment, He opens what the enemy has shut, and just as a key needs to be positioned correctly in the keyhole for a door to open, you also need to be well-aligned so that God can have free course through you.

Your womb is God's special vehicle to birth His will, and even if you don't have a physical womb, God still has spare parts in heaven. In fact, He might not even need a womb to convey His miracle children to the earth! Don't limit God to what you have or don't have. Know His will, align with Him, and watch Him use you as a vehicle to bring Kingdom kids to the earth.

After Hannah aligned her desires with God's will, He opened her womb and caused her to birth His prophet, Samuel. (1 Samuel 1:19). Don't allow your misalignment to keep you in a shutdown state. Cooperate with God in all He has commanded you, and watch Him do what He is a specialist at doing: Opening what no man can shut.

God is the Master Key that opens, and no man can shut. The Master Key will work in your favour in Jesus' name.

PRAYER

1. Lord, I thank you because you are Great, and nothing is hard for you to do. I give you all my worship because you continue to show me favour and increase my strength. Lord Jesus, thank you for opening my womb, empowering it to conceive and making it ready to carry my babies. Hallelujah

2. My Lord Jesus, thank You for Your special plan to make me a vehicle for Your purpose to find expression on the earth. My children and I are for signs and wonder, and we testify to Your unfailing power at opening closed wombs and bypassing no wombs (Isaiah 8:18). Thank You because the channels of my spirit open up to God, and His glory is revealed through me. Amen.

3. In the name of Jesus, everything blocking my womb is destroyed in Jesus name. Every strange object in my womb by whatever name is called, whether it is fibroid or cyst, is completely destroyed in Jesus' name. Whatever God has not planted in me (insert your name) is uprooted in Jesus' name.

4. I decree that my womb is open, fertile, able to conceive, carry to term and deliver safely in Jesus' name. Every tubal spasm, fibroid, endometriosis, cyst, and inflammation is reversed in Jesus' name. I am healed by the stripes of Jesus.

5. My body is the temple of God and is whole and healthy in Jesus' name. God has remembered me for good. I will sing a new song and dance for joy. Like Hannah, God has opened my womb. It's my season of celebration.

I will rejoice and be glad in Jesus' name.

6. My womb is opened in Jesus' name. No one can shut the door you have opened.

7. This is the report of the Lord. I am fruitful, and I multiply. I am carrying my babies. God has looked upon me with favour and has opened my womb. I am a mother of a lovely baby boy, baby girl, twins, triplets, quadruplets etc. I conceive this year, I carry to term and deliver safely in Jesus' name. Amen!!! My husband will carry our babies in Jesus' name. Amen!

GOD HAS REMEMBERED ME

TEXT: PSALM 25:6

REFLECTION:

Can God forget you if a mother cannot forget her suckling child?

Remember me, Lord, when you show favour to your people. Visit us with your deliverance. Psalm 106:4

A lump of clay once felt rejected, neglected and abandoned because the potter had kept it aside. Day after day, it cried for attention and whined to anyone who listened that it was useless. Nights were the hardest because it cried itself to sleep as it watched other lumps of clay transform into beautiful vessels. From its hidden place in a corner, it didn't know that the potter had grand plans for it – plans to make it a silver cup only fit for the best of kings.

Hannah must have felt forgotten when she went year after year to Shiloh with no tangible proof of her devotion. I cannot even imagine Elizabeth's pain, who had to wait years and years before her promise came.

You also might think that God has forgotten your labour, service and sacrifices. Like that lump of clay, you might feel other women have it better than you. If you think this way, stop listening to the devil's lies. God doesn't forget: He never does. When you understand that you are not forgotten, you begin to see God's involvement in all that concerns you. You are not forgotten. You are loved, chosen and watched over.

Your waiting is not because God has forgotten you but because He has remembered you. He is behind the scenes right now, working everything for your good. He is putting together every pain, tear, and sorrow and turning them into an avalanche of joy and glory. He is cooking up your miracle in the best of heaven's pots so that all that looks at you will see His fingerprints upon your life.

You are not forgotten because God has engraved you on the palms of His hands. (Isaiah 49:16). The One who took the time to number every strand of hair on your head has not forgotten (Luke 12:17).

He framed your face, and He remembers you. You are engraved on His mind.

More than a mother is deeply attached to her suckling child; God is attached to you. His watchful eyes are ever on you.

If God forgot you for a split second, the devil would destroy you in less than a quarter of a split second. You are always on God's mind. (Psalm 115:12).

PRAYER

1. Thank You, Jesus, because I am always remembered, never forgotten. Thank You for Your good thoughts towards me. You work behind the scenes, even when I can't feel or see it. I trust You and know that You will always remember me for good. Thank You for loving me, Lord Jesus.

2. Lord Jesus, let me always know you are with me so I will never be afraid or doubt your promises. My Lord and my God, please keep my heart still.

3. I declare, that daily the mercies of God are new towards me. At the breaking of each day, I am reminded of God's love. When I was still a sinner, Jesus loved me. Even now, I am loved. I am not waiting because God hates me or wants to punish me. I am waiting so my faith can be strengthened. I am waiting because God has reserved the best for me.

4. The same God who remembered Sarah, Hannah, Rebecca, Elizabeth, and Mary has remembered me. God cannot forget; He is not man. I am remembered.

5. God has remembered me for good. I will sing a new song and dance for joy. Like Hannah, God has opened my womb. It's my season of celebration. I will rejoice and be glad in Jesus' name.

6. I will continue to declare the promises of God. I will remember the Word of God because it never fails. I will hope in the Lord because those that look to Him remain

radiant. My heart is set on the Lord, and I will carry my own testimony.

7. This is the report of the Lord. I am fruitful, and I multiply. I am carrying my babies. God has looked upon me with favour and has opened my womb. I am a mother of a lovely baby boy, baby girl, twins, triplets, quadruplets etc. I conceive this year, I carry to term and deliver safely in Jesus' name. Amen!!! My husband will carry our babies in Jesus' name. Amen!

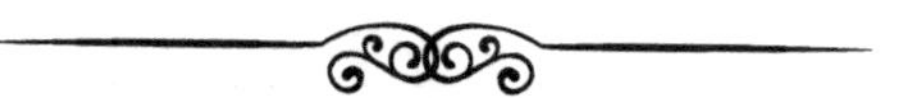

STRENGTHEN ME, O GOD

TEXT: ISAIAH 40:29

REFLECTION:

How desperate are you for God's strength?

But he answered me, "My grace is always more than enough for you, and my power finds its full expression through your weakness." So I will celebrate my weakness, for when I'm weak, I sense more deeply the mighty power of Christ living in me. 2 Corinthians 12:9.

Waiting is tough, especially for a waiting mother. The disappointment of seeing your monthly period, the pregnancy symptoms that are not real, the weight of enduring conversations about children, the loss of interest in sex etc, can be overwhelming. Waiting can be weighty.

Guess what? God has not called us to be supermen who bear their own weight. God wants to carry the burden for you. He wants to wipe your tears, be there for you and take away every yoke, but you must surrender.

When my Father-in-the-Lord lost his dear son in 2021, he was in great pain and sorrow. Nothing and no one could comfort him. One of his spiritual daughters said to him, " Daddy, let God carry you.' My dearest sister, let God carry you. I say the same thing to you. God can carry your weight and pain and carry you as well.

God's strength doesn't come into full play until man's strength gives way. God didn't get involved as long as Sarah knew how to position her maid to bear children for her. God's hands were tied as long as Hannah wanted a child to show Peninnah that she could conceive. If you still know how to work things out in your wisdom, God will wait on the sidelines until you are ready to relinquish control.

God wants to make His strength available to you as you go from one season to another, but are you desperate enough for His invasion? God doesn't look for weaklings; He looks for weakness. And weakness is when you are wise enough not to manipulate things in your favour. It is when you are ready to wait until God shows up. When you don't have alternatives to God - when you surrender completely- He shows up.

Beloved, if you have exhausted all your options and have come up empty, rejoice because God is about to flood you with His life-giving power. If you are weary, God's strength is sufficient to carry you through. Just as Sarah received divine strength to conceive, you, too, will experience the full expression of God's mighty power.

Will you let God carry you from today? Can you surrender completely to Jesus?

PRAYER

1. Thank you, Jesus, for carrying me. Thank you for always being there, loving me and caring for me. Thank you for protecting me from everything and anything that can break my mind. Thank you for your love; your Love is far better than life. Thank you, Jesus.

2. Lord, I receive strength in my inner man. I receive the strength to pray and not be weary, to believe against all hope, to serve my husband, to love those who misunderstand us, to see just as you see and hear just as you hear in Jesus' name.

3. In Jesus' name, I receive the strength to rejoice with those who rejoice. The joy of the Lord is my Strength. I receive the strength to pursue my purpose and fulfil it. I am strengthened to run my race and finish it in Jesus' name. My life will not shut down. I am blooming every day.

4. I am infused with God's Holy power to manifest joy even in this waiting season and prosper in all I do. My life will continue to flourish in Jesus' name. My home will overflow with God's blessings and treasures in Jesus' name.

5. Lord, I receive the strength to pray until my blessing comes. I receive the strength to trust you and not be weary. I receive the strength to bind what must be bound and lose what must be loosed in Jesus' name.

6. Lord, I receive Your strength to conceive and carry my seed to term. I will not miscarry what You have given me in Jesus'

name. God quickens my body to conceive supernaturally in Jesus' name. I have the strength to conceive in Jesus' name.

7. This is the report of the Lord. I am fruitful, and I multiply. I am carrying my babies. God has looked upon me with favour and has opened my womb. I am a mother of a lovely baby boy, baby girl, twins, triplets, quadruplets etc. I conceive this year, I carry to term and deliver safely in Jesus' name. Amen!!! My husband will carry our babies in Jesus' name. Amen!

I CAN SEE, AND I WILL CARRY MY CHILDREN

TEXT: 1 SAMUEL 1:27

REFLECTION:

What can you see?

For all the land which you see I will give to you and to your posterity forever. Genesis 13:15 AMPC

What can you see, beloved? A house full of children or an empty house? A womb with children or a barren womb? Life is spiritual, and whatever you see in your mind becomes your reality. After Lot left Abram, God asked Abram what he could see. 'Open your eyes, look around,' God told him. 'Look north, south, east and west. Genesis 13:14 MSG.

Faith is seeing what God sees about you and believing it. It is seeing with your spiritual eyes what is invisible to your natural eyes. When you see your life through God's eyes, you will speak and act according to what has been revealed. Faith does not make sense; it makes Miracles.

Faith is how we make tangible what was not existing before.

Don't focus on what others have said because their words, thoughts or reports don't count. Look unto Jesus and see what He sees.

I want you to create a folder on your phone and save pictures of babies. If you love twins, boys or girls, save their pictures. If you want triplets, then save their pictures. Look for things that look like your future. Buy some baby items and put them where you can see them often. Train your mind to see the possibility you already know in your Spirit.

When I was trusting God for twin babies, I downloaded hundreds of pictures and sowed seeds for them. I gave a certain amount every month as my faith seed. This was long before I met my husband, and God honoured my faith.

Now proclaim this boldly, *'I can see my children, and I will carry them. I will have what I see.'*

Joshua and Caleb saw that they could conquer the Canaanites and enter the Promised Land, and they had what they saw. Though your babies have tarried, don't stop seeing them. Soon, they will manifest in the flesh.

PRAYER

1. Thank You, Jesus, for a new sight. I see what You see and have what I see. I am a fruitful vine, and my children surround my table. My thoughts, feelings and actions align with what I see in the Spirit. I can see my children, and I carry them, not only in my womb but in my hands too. Amen.

2. I declare that my Spirit is charged with fresh, mountain-defying faith in Jesus' name. I am empowered to see through the eyes of faith in Jesus' name. I receive the same faith that showed Moses a way where there was no way and showed Jesus a living man even when Lazarus was dead for four days. I receive great faith in Jesus' name!

3. My heart and mind will not be broken and filled with hopeless thoughts. The light of God invades my heart and thoughts in Jesus' name. Light has come, and darkness must flee in Jesus' name. I bring into captivity every thought that is contending with God in my life in Jesus' name.

4. Mention the names of your children. Call their names and declare that you see them. Carry them in your hands and dance around your house. Break free from fear and hopelessness in Jesus' name. Dare to believe!!!

5. I see the Lord working it out for my good. I can see the hand of the Lord turning in my favour. I can see the Lord making a way for me. I can see the Lord bringing in my miracles. I see the Lord fighting all my battles. I see the Lord comforting me in Jesus' name. Hallelujah!

6. I see the doctor's report turned around. I see men and women rejoicing with me. I see my big tummy filled with my babies. I see my husband rejoicing. My mother and his mother are dancing for joy. I see the Lord has done it!!! Hallelujah!

7. This is the report of the Lord. I am fruitful, and I multiply. I am carrying my babies. God has looked upon me with favour and has opened my womb. I am a mother of a lovely baby boy, baby girl, twins, triplets, quadruplets etc. I conceive this year, I carry to term and deliver safely in Jesus' name. Amen!!! My husband will carry our babies in Jesus' name. Amen!

I CANCEL EVERY NEGATIVE DREAM

TEXT: PSALM 27:1

REFLECTION:

What are you permitting in your space?

Submit yourself therefore to God. Resist the devil and he will flee from you. James 4:7 KJV

Your dream life is as real as your life here on earth. Humans are active only when awake, but spiritual activities continue even when men are asleep. (Job 33:15-18).

Your body may sleep, but your spirit is powerfully active and exposed to the spirit realm. Where you belong in the Spirit realm will determine the kind of activities you attract.

Sometimes dreams can reflect our deepest thoughts, but most times, they are signals God is calling us to pay attention to.

Some people were attacked in their dreams and woke up with parts of their bodies maimed. Some people are struggling to conceive because of demonic activities that occur in their sleep. A woman who miscarries her pregnancy every time she has sex in her dream is under demonic attack.

I have profited too many times to count from dreams. God wants to show you things in your dreams as much as He speaks to you in your thoughts.

Dreams are vehicles that convey messages to us, and just as God gives dreams, the devil gives dreams too. Sometimes, God can confirm His Word, instruct or warn you through dreams. When you have dreams, don't shove them aside because they can contain critical messages. When God gives you a warning dream, it comes with grace, hope and a way of escape when you take heed.

The following steps are how you should respond to your dreams;

I.   **Give thanks.** No matter what you see in your dream, make sure you give God praise. Even if the devil runs mad, God is still God. Thanksgiving breaks the devil's stronghold, so he cannot influence your interpretation of the dream. It keeps your mind at peace, enthrones God and gives you the right perspective. A bad dream can be a revelation or warning from God. It is not always an attack.

You will only know if you give thanks. You will only know

when your mind is at rest.

II. **Ask God for understanding**. Ask, and you will receive. (John 16:24). Ask and Wait on God for a clear understanding of your dreams. God is more eager to give you clarity than you. While waiting for God to give meaning to the dream, cancel any negative interpretation from the dream if it is a bad dream. Speak peace over your life.

III. **Don't get so fixated on the dream**. Don't idolize the dream. The dream may be one part of a message. The other part may be in a sermon or a conversation. Your attention and focus should be on God.

IV. **Leave the dream if you have prayed and there is no understanding or instruction from God**. God knows how to speak to you. Don't worry about it so the enemy does not fill your mind with the wrong ideas. Write it in your journal when understanding or complete understanding comes; you can always refer to it.

V.   **You can also share the dream with a mature believer who is not desperate to impress you** - Someone who is prophetically inclined and will pray with and for you.

Your dream is purified and sanctified to God in Jesus' name. You will dream the dreams of God in Jesus' name.

PRAYER

1. Father, I thank You for an active and pure dream life. I recognize that You communicate to me through visions and dreams. I thank You for speaking to me in my dreams and always giving me the understanding of what is revealed.

2. I decree that my dream portal is covered by the blood of Jesus. The enemy has no access to my dreams in Jesus' name. I will no longer see or hear things God does not ordain in Jesus' name. I will no longer have nightmares in Jesus' name. My sleep is sweet and restful in Jesus' name. (Proverbs 3:24).

3. I nullify every satanic agenda to deceive me and fill my life with lies in Jesus' name. I will not dream the dreams of the devil in Jesus' name. My lying down is unto the Lord. My bed is sanctified and a place of worship to God in Jesus' name. Even in my sleep, I fellowship with God. His holy Presence surrounds me in Jesus' name.

4. I stand in my authority as God's child and cancel every negative dream in Jesus' name. Amen. I nullify every satanic dream that continues to reoccur in my life in Jesus' name. I nullify every satanic attack targeted at my dreams in Jesus' name. I declare I am victorious in all my dreams in Jesus' name.

5. I cover my husband with the blood of Jesus. He will not dream evil dreams or be drawn into demonic conspiracy via his dreams in Jesus' name. My husband is full of divine discernment and has supernatural clarity in Jesus' name.

6. From today, I dream the dreams of God in Jesus' name. The things that are important to my life are revealed to me in Jesus' name. I will no longer forget my dreams in Jesus' name. I have an understanding of my dreams in Jesus' name. Every dream relevant to my life that the enemy stole from me is now restored in Jesus' name.

7. This is the report of the Lord. I am fruitful, and I multiply. I am carrying my babies. God has looked upon me with favour and has opened my womb. I am a mother of a lovely baby boy, baby girl, twins, triplets, quadruplets etc. I conceive this year, I carry to term and deliver safely in Jesus' name. Amen!!! My husband will carry our babies in Jesus' name. Amen!

I UPROOT WHATEVER GOD HAS NOT PLANTED IN MY BODY AND MY HUSBAND'S BODY

TEXT: MATTHEW 15:13

REFLECTION:

What stranger needs to leave your body or your husband's body?

See, I have this day set thee over the nations and over the kingdoms, to root out, and to pull down, and to destroy, and to throw down, to build, and to plant. Jeremiah 1:10 KJV

The enemy steals by introducing evil elements, which are his weapons. The devil steals peace by planting worry. He steals prosperity by planting greed, fear or lust in the heart. He steals good health by planting sicknesses and diseases. He steals purity by planting lustful thoughts.

You are responsible for uprooting everything God has not planted in your life. The power to bind and loose is yours to exercise.

When a woodcutter wants to cut a tree, he doesn't cut it from the branches or stem; he aims for the root. And when a farmer plants, he doesn't joke with weeds - He roots them out mercilessly because he knows what they are capable of. Anything God has not planted in your body is a weed and a stranger and should not be spared. Whatever God has not planted or authored in your husband's body shouldn't be pampered too.

As a woman, you are a watchman, and you have authority in Jesus to remove anything He has not planted in your space. Whether fibroid, cysts, blocked tubes, tumours or whatever name it has, the name of Jesus supersedes them all. (Philippians 2:10). Use the name of Jesus to uproot them.

Put the axe of God's Word against their roots. Be ruthless in uprooting every stranger in your body. Be consistent in your attack against everything God has not planted, and don't stop proclaiming your victory until it manifests in the natural.

Whatever you permit stays permitted. Whatever you disallow is completely disallowed. You are royalty, and Heaven backs your decree. (Matthew 16:19).

PRAYER

1. Thank you, Father, for you have never lost a battle. Thank you, Jesus, because in your name, every knee must bow, and every tongue must confess you as Lord. Jehovah Nissi, you are my Banner, my Covering, my Fortress. By your everlasting Arm, I go from victory to victory in Jesus' name.

2. In the name of Jesus, everything that God has not planted in my life, my body and that of my husband is uprooted in Jesus' name. Every stranger is cast out in Jesus' name.

3. Today, I speak to every part of my body and my husband's body, hear God's Word and function according to God's original design. I root out every stranger (mention them) in our bodies and pull down every high thing in our bodies and lives that has exalted itself against the knowledge of Christ. (2 Corinthians 10:5). We walk in total victory over every strange ailment, condition, or disease in Jesus' name. Amen.

4. Whatever I permitted in my body through negative utterances, past sexual relationships, occultic practices in the time of ignorance, and ungodly things my parents did on my behalf to protect me are all destroyed in Jesus' name. I renounce them in the mighty name of Jesus!!!

5. By the Arm of the Lord, every strange thing in my body and my husband's body is ejected in Jesus' name. My body is God's temple, and strangers are prohibited and banned from gaining access. I refuse to accommodate anything that does not glorify God in Jesus' name.

6. From today, I am free from strange ailments and manifestations in my body in Jesus' name. I bring an end to every demonic encounter in Jesus' name. My body is blessed and sanctified unto God in Jesus' name.

7. This is the report of the Lord. I am fruitful, and I multiply. I am carrying my babies. God has looked upon me with favour and has opened my womb. I am a mother of a lovely baby boy, baby girl, twins, triplets, quadruplets etc. I conceive this year, I carry to term and deliver safely in Jesus' name. Amen!!! My husband will carry our babies in Jesus' name. Amen!

I BREAK EVERY NEGATIVE GENERATIONAL PATTERN

TEXT: MARK 14:22-25

REFLECTION:

How can you stop negative patterns and start positive ones?

Behold, I will do a new thing; now it shall spring forth; shall ye not know it? I will even make a way in the wilderness, and rivers in the desert. Isaiah 43:19 KJV.

Some believers believe negative generational patterns cannot manifest in their lives. Indeed, a believer cannot be cursed because they are in Christ, and Christ cannot be cursed.

However, if a believer fails to exercise their authority, the enemy will bring the affliction of their father or mother on them. The devil is no respecter of persons or anointing; he only fears the Spoken Word. He fears believers who exercise their authority. He only fears believers who know their authority and use this authority powerfully. He is a bully, and he is willing to take his chances with you irrespective of the number of years you have been saved or how much you love God.

Galatians 4:1 (KJV) Now I say, That the heir, as long as he is a child, differeth nothing from a servant, though he be Lord of all;

The Bible says a believer who is a child of God, anointed, elevated, empowered and already victorious, is not different from a slave if he is a child in spiritual matters. A slave is subject to the limitations of this world. Why? Because he is a child.
If you remain a child in spiritual things, though you are anointed and blessed, your life will say otherwise.

This is why Jesus gave us the power to bind and loose. Jesus knew for a certainty that our business here on earth would include binding and loosing because life is warfare.

Matthew 16:19 (KJV) And I will give unto thee the keys of the kingdom of heaven: and whatsoever thou shalt bind on earth shall be bound in heaven: and whatsoever thou shalt loose on earth shall be loosed in heaven.

You must have a victorious mindset and ensure your declarations are victorious because as you think in your heart, so are you(Proverbs

23:7). The first battleground is your mind. What you know in your head must frame your mind and colour your thoughts. You must hold deep convictions about what God says about you.

A pattern is a recurring cycle that can be positive or negative. David created a positive pattern of following God and set a standard that God used to measure the kings after him. He also set a negative pattern of unbridled lust when he took Uriah's wife, which his son, Solomon, inherited and amplified.

Abraham waited for Isaac, and Isaac also waited for Jacob and Esau. This pattern of waiting for children also affected Jacob because his beloved Rachel had to wait a while before Joseph was born.

What patterns did you meet in your family? What patterns did your husband meet in his? Jesus set a new pattern for us when He gave His body and blood to His disciples as a token of the new covenant. Holy Communion is not a lifeless or mindless ritual but a gateway into the covenant of life and peace.

Identify the negative patterns in your family (yours and your husband's) and take the communion continuously as you engage God to break them. Do this with understanding, and ask the Lord to reveal negative patterns you are unaware of. As you destroy negative patterns through the blood and flesh of Jesus, create new, positive ones. Engage the blood and flesh of Jesus against every negative cycle, and use them to raise new altars.

PRAYER

(Say this prayer for and with your husband.)

1. Father of Light, I thank you for being good and kind. Thank you, Jesus, for saving me from the power of darkness and giving me victory over every power of the enemy. Thank you, for whatever is not in Christ has no power over me.

2. Today, I decree and declare that I am free from every satanic attack. I will not inherit the limitations of my father or mother. I am in Christ, old things have passed away, and all things are made new. By the blood of Jesus, I have escaped every evil in my father or mother's bloodline. The blood of Jesus is my DNA. The enemy has no legal ground to afflict me in Jesus' name.

3. I rebuke every false mindset, disillusion, burden and presence confronting my fruitfulness in Jesus' name. No weapon formed against me will prosper.

4. I come out of every negative pattern I permitted in ignorance because I thought it was natural. I break free from every satanic mindset in Jesus' name. I renounce every sickness or disease, or negative condition; I called mine. They are not mine; they are uprooted from my body and life in Jesus' name.

5. I destroy every soul tie the enemy is seeking to enforce against me. Every demonic alliance to oppress and destroy me is completely destroyed in Jesus' name. Let your mercy prevail over my family; my father's house, my mother's

house and my husband's house, in Jesus' name. Let Your mercy prevail in Jesus' name. Psalm 51:1-2

6. As I take the body and blood of Jesus, I destroy every negative pattern and cycle in my ancestry and my husband's ancestry. Together, we raise new altars and positive patterns of fruitfulness, abundance, no delays or denials, righteousness, and (add others) in Jesus' name. Amen.

7. This is the report of the Lord. I am fruitful, and I multiply. I am carrying my babies. God has looked upon me with favour and has opened my womb. I am a mother of a lovely baby boy, baby girl, twins, triplets, quadruplets etc. I conceive this year, I carry to term and deliver safely in Jesus' name. Amen!!! My husband will carry our babies in Jesus' name. Amen!

LORD, HONOUR YOUR WORD IN MY LIFE

TEXT: LEVITICUS 26:9

REFLECTION:

What areas do you want God to honour His Word in your life?

I bow down before your divine Presence and bring you my deepest worship as I experience your tender love and your living truth. For Your Word and the fame of Your name have been magnified above all else. Psalm 138:2 TPT

God is bound to honour His Word. He has esteemed His Word far above His name. He has decreed that His Word will not return to Him void. (Isaiah 55:11). He is the Monarch of Heaven, and His Word is law.

The easiest way to sail in an ocean is to sail in the direction of the wind, not against it. Any ship that sails against the wind might not survive if the wind is boisterous—bringing your complaints before God is sailing against the wind of His principles. He only has respect for His Word, name and covenant.

God will not honour what He has not said, and if you want to hasten your miracle, always remind Him of His Word. Mary told the Lord that it should be unto her according to His Word, not her emotions, ambitions, or the reports of others. (Luke 1:38).

You have a responsibility to fill your heart, mind and life with the Word of God. He cannot honour His Word in your life if it is simply in your head. The Word of God is honoured when it goes forth. Make sure you are constantly speaking and declaring the Word of God. As you do so, the honour of God will rest on your life and all that you cherish in Jesus' name.

Speak God's Word to Him in prayers. Remind Him of His promises as you praise and worship. Tell Him of the decrees He has made concerning you. Don't stop speaking His Word until everything about you flows in the direction of His will. When you hold God by His Word, dead things spring to life, and new things happen. Miracles happen when God honours His Word in your life. Ask the Lord to honour His Word in your life, and He will.

PRAYER

1. Father, I give you all the praise and glory, you have highly esteemed Your Word above Your name.
Psalms 138:2 (KJV) I *will worship toward thy holy temple, and praise thy name for thy lovingkindness and for thy truth: for thou hast magnified thy word above all thy name.*

2. Father, I decree that your Word is potent in my life and my life is a powerful reflection of your Word.
Isaiah 55:11 (KJV*) So shall my word be that goeth forth out of my mouth: it shall not return unto me void, but it shall accomplish that which I please, and it shall prosper in the thing whereto I sent it.*

3. Lord, every Prophetic word spoken over me according to Your will be speedily fulfilled in Jesus' name. Let your Word be fulfilled in my life. Father, I declare that my prayers are answered. I rejoice that my prayers are answered speedily in Jesus' name.

4. I hold firmly to Your Word, which You have magnified above all else. Lord, your Word is honoured in my life and family in Jesus' name. Amen. I will see the Word of God manifest in my life and marriage in Jesus' name.

5. Father, I repent from every act of disobedience that may have caused the delay of the fulfilment of your Word in my life. Holy Spirit, please show me any area I need to realign with God. If unforgiveness in my heart has hindered God from

moving in my life, Lord, I repent totally from it in Jesus' name.

6. Father, let only your Word be true in my life, and all other voices be lies in Jesus' name. I stand only on your Word because all other ground is sinking sand.

7. This is the report of the Lord. I am fruitful, and I multiply. I am carrying my babies. God has looked upon me with favour and has opened my womb. I am a mother of a lovely baby boy, baby girl, twins, triplets, quadruplets etc. I conceive this year, I carry to term and deliver safely in Jesus' name. Amen!!! My husband will carry our babies in Jesus' name. Amen!

I AM ANOINTED TO BE FRUITFUL

TEXT: GENESIS 17:6

REFLECTION:

Are you ready for the fresh oil of fruitfulness?

But my horn shalt thou exalt like the horn of an unicorn: I shall be anointed with fresh oil. Psalm 92:10 KJV

God, in the beginning, blessed man and called him fruitful. God designed and empowered both man and woman to be fruitful. Barrenness is not normal because, in the beginning, it was not so. You are blessed, empowered and anointed to be fruitful in your body and in all things.

After Hannah's wordless prayer in Shiloh and Eli's blessings, something happened that made her well-positioned for her miracle baby. She came there with a sorrowful spirit but left there joyful. The Bible records that she went her way, ate and was no longer sad. (1 Samuel 1:18). Hannah received the anointing of fruitfulness after she laid down her sorrow and became joyful. Joy positions you for this anointing because joy is a fetcher of good things. With joy, you draw water out of the wells of salvation. Isaiah 12:3.

The anointing is the empowerment to shake off every limitation and step into all God has given you.

The oil is symbolic of the anointing, and oil produces ease. It also facilitates speed and removes tension and friction. Oil also removes shame and makes the face shine.
'And wine that makes glad the heart of man, and oil to make his face to shine, and bread which strengthens man's heart.' Psalm 104:15.

Oil also overflows, and the overflowing anointing of fruitfulness is God's portion for you. It is not just for you but for everyone that comes in contact with you. God is releasing fresh oil upon you, but you need joy to access it. Let go of your heaviness and sorrow, and dance before God today.

Proclaim this loudly and boldly, and let the devil hear, *'My head is lifted like that of a unicorn, above shame and sorrow. I will no longer know sorrow, delay and shame because I have traded my sorrow for joy and dryness for fruitfulness.'*

Just spend quality time basking in God's Presence today as He releases this anointing upon you.

A fresh anointing for fruitfulness is resting upon you today in Jesus' name.

PRAYER

1. Father, I thank you because you have called me fruitful from the beginning, and no one can defeat your Word. Thank you for making me and anointing me to be fruitful. I thank you, Lord, for your Word comes alive in me today, and I bear fruits in my body and all things in Jesus' name.

2. I am anointed with fresh oil – the oil of gladness and fruitfulness. My head doesn't lack oil, and I am fruitful on every side. As a fruitful vine, my cup overflows, and everyone that comes in contact with me becomes fruitful. Amen.

3. I am fruitful in my body, a joyful mother of children. I am fruitful in all my endeavours and do not know vain labour in Jesus' name. All the works of my hands are blessed in Jesus' name.

4. From today, everything in my body is quickened to be fruitful in Jesus' name. In Jesus' name, I uproot anything that shouldn't be in my body. If parts of my body have grown weak or died, I speak life over them in Jesus' name.

5. I am not barren, nor do I miscarry my young. I have the blessing of the Lord. God has blessed me with blessings from above, from the earth and of the womb. I am blessed in Jesus' name. (Genesis 49:25).

6. Whatever was said or done to hinder my fruitfulness has now been undone in Jesus' name. I come in the name of the

Lord and cancel every attack on my fruitfulness in Jesus'
name. I speak peace over every attack and storm in my life
and family in Jesus' name.

7. This is the report of the Lord. I am fruitful, and I multiply. I
    am carrying my babies. God has looked upon me with favour
    and has opened my womb. I am a mother of a lovely baby
    boy, baby girl, twins, triplets, quadruplets etc. I conceive
    this year, I carry to term and deliver safely in Jesus' name.
    Amen!!! My husband will carry our babies in Jesus' name.
    Amen!

I REBUKE THE SPIRIT OF DEATH

TEXT: HEBREWS 2:15

REFLECTION:

Where has death reigned in your body or family?

Our God is the God who will make us free. The Lord our God will save us from death. Psalm 68:20 Easy English.

The work of the enemy is to steal, kill and destroy. He loves to bring death to the things that glorify God. You must not allow him to spread death in your body or home. You are designed to bring glory to God. Jesus gave us Life; He gave us abundant life. You have an abundant life. The very Life of God is in you.

You have the Zoe Life, and it is the Life that swallows death in victory. Hallelujah!

Death is not only present when someone takes his last breath; it is present when there is no life. When things don't function as God intended, death reigns. And when you suffer lack in one area or the other, or you don't have all that God desires for you to have, death is hiding somewhere. Jesus' death has set you free from death of any kind. He died on the cross so that you may have life.

Whether it is a non-functioning organ or a situation that doesn't conform to God's will, you don't have to permit death in your space. Jesus wants you to have Life – abundant, overflowing and more-than-enough Life.

Whenever you see death at work, reverse and rebuke its effects by standing on the Life in God's word. Remember, death and life are in the power of your tongue.(Proverbs 18:21). Use your tongue to speak life to your womb, life and family. Speak life into all that concerns you. And be careful not to counter your words with negative and death-like thoughts. Fill your mind with the life in God's word, and let your mouth proclaim what your mind sees.

It doesn't matter how your body feels, what the doctors are saying or not saying, what you have seen in dreams; you will live long in good health and sound mind in Jesus' name.

PRAYER

1. Thank you, Jesus, for giving me Life abundantly. Thank you for the river of Life flowing in me and everything I touch. Thank you, Lord, for I will live and not die. Thank you, Jesus, for your Life reigns in my body. Hallelujah!

2. I am alive in Christ Jesus, and I live, move and have my being in Him (Acts 17:28). I speak life to my womb, and all that concerns me, and I enjoy abundant life. I decree that death has no place in me or around me. Amen.

3. The gates of hell will not prevail over my life, body, husband, marriage and everything that pertains to me. I decree that darkness cannot prevail. Light shines!!! Where the Light of God is, there is Life. I decree that light prevails in my body, my husband's body and my family in Jesus' name.

4. Women receive their dead back to life. (Hebrews 11:35). I receive back to life everything that has died or is dying in my life in Jesus' name. Whatever failed in my body, my h husband's body and our lives; by the same power that raised Jesus from the dead, that quickening power brings everything dead or dying back to life in Jesus' name.

5. The blood of Jesus speaks!! It speaks life, peace, mercy and Divine order in Jesus' name. By the blood of Jesus, I decree that death, infertility, lack, premature birth, and miscarriage have passed over my home in Jesus' name. The blood of Jesus is a covering over my in Jesus' name.

6.   The last time I wept over dead things in my life is the last
      time I will ever weep in Jesus' name.
      The power of God rests upon me, and death is cancelled in my
      life in Jesus' name. Everything that died is restored to me with
      double compensation in Jesus' name.
7.   This is the report of the Lord. I am fruitful, and I multiply.
      I am carrying my babies. God has looked upon me with favour
      and has opened my womb. I am a mother of a lovely baby boy,
      baby girl, twins, triplets, quadruplets etc. I conceive this year,
      I carry to term and deliver safely in Jesus' name. Amen!!! My
      husband will carry our babies in Jesus' name. Amen!

MY BODY IS QUICKENED

TEXT: 1 CORINTHIANS 15:45

REFLECTION:

As a life-giving spirit, how can you live in the fullness of your spiritual reality?

Yes, God raised Jesus to life! And since God's Spirit of Resurrection lives in you, he will also raise your dying body to life by the same spirit that breathes life into you! Romans 8:11 TPT

When Jesus died, it seemed as though God's plans of salvation had been buried, sealed, and eternally forgotten, but little did the devil know that his worst was about to become man's greatest gain. God's strategy to raise Jesus from the dead was to send the

Spirit of resurrection, the Holy Spirit, to quicken Him from the dead.

This is the same plan He has for you. The Holy Spirit has been given to you to quicken your body and make you a partaker of God's fullness - He is your gateway to the fullness of life.

You must understand you are a supernatural being full of the Holy Ghost and He is the Holy Spirit of God.You are not ordinary. You are full of life-giving power. You are not subject to the law of death like others; you are powerfully exempted.

Say after me, *'I am exempted from every evil attack in Jesus' name.'*

The power of the Holy Ghost quickened the body of Abraham and Sarah so that though they were old and past the age of childbearing, they were able to birth a son. Nothing is hard for God to do.

Life is in your body. If you use your authority in the name of Jesus, you will bring to life whatever is dying in your body.

Today, spend some time praying in the Spirit and allow the Spirit of resurrection to stir up the waters of life in you. Your body is quickened to bear fruit and bring forth speedily. When the Resurrection and the Life visited Lazarus' tomb, a 4-day-old, stinking, dead body sprang to life. (John 11:25). Believe in Him because nothing remains impossible for those who believe.

You should also know that healthy living is crucial. Eating right, fasting the right way, resting well, exercising well, and not consuming harmful substances help your body do what God has commanded it to do. Faith without works is void. When we pray but fail to do our part, we limit God in our lives.

I know God, who put this book in your hands, is about to do something powerful in your life.

Your testimony will be beautiful and loud in Jesus' name.

PRAYER

1. Thank you, Father of Life. Thank you for your quickening power. Thank you for giving me life abundantly. I have the same power that raised dry bones and Lazarus from the dead, the same power that healed the woman with the issue of blood and the men with leprosy. (Romans 8:11). Thank you for that same power is at work in me in Jesus' name.

2. My body is quickened because the Spirit of resurrection lives in me. I am alive, and every body organ functions to full capacity. The quickening power of God surges through me, and my womb receives life and carries children to full term. Amen.

3. (Put your hand on the part of your body where you are sick and pray). I command every arrow of witchcraft in my body to be uprooted in Jesus' name. I am healed from every satanic attack in Jesus' name.

4. Every evil by whatever name called anaemia, leukaemia, haemophilia etc., hiding in my blood is flushed out in Jesus' name. My body rejects everything that is not of God. No weapon formed against me will prosper in Jesus' name. (Isaiah 54:17).

5. By Your stripes, I am healed. I am free from every sickness and disease in Jesus' name. My body is cleansed from every infirmity, sickness and disease in Jesus' name. You sent Your Word, and Your Word has healed me in Jesus' name. (Psalms 107:20).

6. If there are doctors or treatments that You would want to use to heal this disease, Lord, I receive guidance from the Holy Spirit on the doctor and treatment You have ordained in

Jesus' name. I receive wisdom and discernment about which treatments to pursue. My body cooperates with God in Jesus' name.

7. This is the report of the Lord. I am fruitful, and I multiply. I am carrying my babies. God has looked upon me with favour and has opened my womb. I am a mother of a lovely baby boy, baby girl, twins, triplets, quadruplets etc. I conceive this year, I carry to term and deliver safely in Jesus' name. Amen!!! My husband will carry our babies in Jesus' name. Amen!

I CANCEL EVERY NEGATIVE UTTERANCE

TEXT: PHILIPPIANS 4:8

REFLECTION:

Why will a lie act like the truth in your life?

Take counsel together, and it shall come to nought; speak the word, and it shall not stand: for God is with us. Isaiah 8:10

People think words are nothing. They feel that the only words that count are those spoken intentionally; even then, people believe some words can be discarded. Well, that's outright ignorance. Words are always powerful! God's Word created the visible world we see today.

Matthew 12:36-37 (KJV) *But I say unto you, That every idle word that men shall speak, they shall give account thereof in the day of judgment.*
For by thy words thou shalt be justified, and by thy words thou shalt be condemned.

Some of us have said things we shouldn't have said in a time of ignorance. Some people placed a curse on themselves in a moment of passion and love.

I remember when I was working at Dove TV. I interviewed a former Occultic Warlord who is now an Evangelist, Joshua Milton Bhlayi. He spoke of how they lured parents through idle conversations that gave their children away so they could have legality over the children in the realm of the spirit.
He spoke of wanting to use a girl for rituals but could not get the girl's mother to make an idle statement. He had to buy gifts for the girl and got her to say she was his wife jokingly. He needed her consent to exert authority over her, and he got it in a careless statement.
All they need is the spoken word. It matters little if you mean it or not.

Esau lost his birthright because of careless and idle talk. He spoke nonchalantly and lost his birthright. It was a simple conversation to him, but Jacob was negotiating his destiny with him.

May we not be ensnared by the words of our mouth in Jesus' name. Some people are victims of the idle words they speak, while some are victims of the words spoken over their lives. Some parents have done things that have limited their children. A man spoke about how he would see a masquerade in his dreams anytime he was about to move to the next level in his business. This went on for years until his father told him during a casual conversation one day that he made sacrifices on him and his siblings' behalf to the family idol, a masquerade that protected them all. This man often gave his father money for the family rite anytime his father was travelling to the village. He had no idea what the money was used for and why his father travelled until that conversation happened. He had to tell his father outrightly that he was not a part of the family rites and stopped paying for the rituals.

You must renounce every word spoken against God's will for your life. Malicious words spoken against you and evil covenants should be cancelled. The things you said that others now hold against you are cancelled in Jesus' name. You must confess and renounce them all.

You must also exercise authority to condemn every tongue that rises against you. (Isaiah 54:17). You can go into heaven's court and shut down every decree or divination against your ability to give birth. Take your place, warrior woman, in heaven's court and proclaim God's decree against everything that doesn't align with God's will for your life.

PRAYER

1. Thank you, Lord, for you are the Living Word. You are the Word, the Word is with you, and the Word is God. Thank you for your Word has prevailed over my life, and all other voices are silenced in Jesus' name. Thank you, Jesus.

2. Father, I decree that only your Word will prevail over my life. Every other voice speaking against my family in the place of judgment is now condemned in Jesus' name. (Isaiah 54:17). I am free from every malicious gang-up and satanic attack in Jesus' name.

3. I renounce every idle word spoken ignorantly that the enemy now seeks to use against me. I reject every word spoken over me that is against the Will of God for my life in Jesus' name.

4. I stand on my spiritual authority to bring to judgment every tongue speaking negatively about me. I decree that every word spoken against me is null and void in Jesus' name. Every negative utterance against me is disannulled. Amen.

5. No enchantment, divination, spell or sorcery can work against me. They are all nullified. Instead, I walk in supernatural wonders in Jesus' name (Numbers 23:23).

6. Today, I speak life, health, abundance, victory, and favour over my life and my husband in Jesus' name. We prosper in all things good and godly in Jesus' name.

7. This is the report of the Lord. I am fruitful, and I multiply. I

am carrying my babies. God has looked upon me with favour and has opened my womb. I am a mother of a lovely baby boy, baby girl, twins, triplets, quadruplets etc. I conceive this year, I carry to term and deliver safely in Jesus' name. Amen!!! My husband will carry our babies in Jesus' name. Amen!

I ACTIVATE EVERY PROPHECY SPOKEN INTO MY LIFE

TEXT: 2 PETER 1:19-21

REFLECTION:

What will hasten the divine prophecies over your life into fulfilment?

This charge I commit unto you, (put your name), according to the prophecies which went before on you, that you by them might war a good warfare. 1 Timothy 1:18

Whenever you receive a prophecy, know that it is a call to war. It is a call to war because satan will do all he can to keep it from happening. He will fight tooth and nail to ensure you don't look like your prophecy. And if he has succeeded in making a mockery out of the words you have received before now, his show is over!

Paul told Timothy to get to war because of the prophecies he had received. You, too, will do the same. You will get those old journals out and reread those jotters. You will write out those prophecies on a plain sheet of paper and paste them in a place where you can see them daily. And you will war over them until you can touch them.

You will war over them in prayers and worship. You will hold them before the Lord and birth them. You will activate every word God has said in His word and those He has spoken through others. And you will not stop warring until you look exactly like your prophecies. Prophecies are not automatic, nor are they gifts from Santa. You must contend for them. No contention, No possession. You must insist on what was spoken over your life.

Sometimes, fertility delay is not about you having children. It's about attacking your faith and distracting you from the future God revealed through His prophets. The enemy wants to use this to sink your faith and your life. Don't let him. Become very aggressive in the Spirit and declare your prophetic destiny.

Open doors always attract opposition (1 Corinthians 16:9). Get up and fight for what is yours. Jesus secured your victory already. Now, enforce it!

Deuteronomy 2:24 (KJV) *Rise ye up, take your journey, and pass over the river Arnon: behold, I have given into thine hand Sihon the Amorite, king of Heshbon, and his land: begin to possess it, and contend with him in battle.*

I encourage you to record the dreams and prophecies you will receive or have received through others. Write them in a journal or create an email for them. Prophecies are powerful weapons for spiritual warfare.

I want you also to remember that you are the first Prophet of your life. If a prophecy does not give you faith, hope and establish you in the love of God, you should not accept it. The essence of prophecy is edification (1 Corinthians 14:3).
You don't have to wait or hire a prophet to receive prophetic insight or declaration. The Holy Ghost is the spirit of prophecy and lives in you. Open your mouth and prophesy over your life.

Prophesy over your life now, *'I am blessed and highly favoured by God and man.'*

PRAYER

1. Thank you, Father, for your Word is true, faithful and powerful. Your Word is my Anchor, Future and Reality. It is unstoppable, unquestionable, unquenchable and indefatigable. I stand secure on your Word because it can never fail.

2. (Read out every prophecy you have ever received in God's word and through others concerning your children. As you read each of them, pray in understanding and the spirit. Activate them in God's presence and keep them alive on the altar of prayer until you can see, touch, smell and hear them.)

3. In the name of Jesus, I decree that the fullness of time has come for the Word of God to manifest in my life. Lord, remember me today and let there be a manifestation of your Word in my life in Jesus' name.

4. I come against every resistance and opposition to my prophetic destiny in Jesus' name. I decree that the spoken Word is established in Jesus' name.

5. I receive Faith for the substance of things I am hoping for, and I have evidence of the unseen blessings God has given me. My faith is increased, helped and enlarged. My faith will not grow weary or weak. God has helped my faith.

6. A new dawn has come. I decree that a new dawn has come. I see it clearly in Jesus' name. It's the dawn of a new day, fulfilled dreams and prophecies. I see manifestations from today in Jesus' name.

7. This is the report of the Lord. I am fruitful, and I multiply. I am carrying my babies. God has looked upon me with favour and has opened my womb. I am a mother of a lovely baby boy, baby girl, twins, triplets, quadruplets etc. I conceive this year, I carry to term and deliver safely in Jesus' name. Amen!!! My husband will carry our babies in Jesus' name. Amen!

DAY 20

THE LORD HEARS ME, AND HE WILL ANSWER ME

TEXT: PSALM 3:4

REFLECTION:

Have you felt like God isn't listening to your prayers recently?

In my distress, I cried unto the Lord, and he heard me. Psalm 120:1

The Bible has repeated stories of people who cried unto God, and He heard them. He didn't only listen to them; He also answered their prayers. God is not a prayer-storing God; He is a prayer-answering God.

And indeed, He hears your prayers as loudly as He hears your thoughts.

Waiting can make you 'feel' like your prayers are not heard. The enemy can begin to play with your mind and give you the impression that God prefers some people more than you, or that God has exempted you from the blessing of having a child, or you must have done something that God is punishing you for, etc. These are some evil thoughts the enemy can begin to plant in your mind; they are all lies! None of the above is scriptural. God is mandated to hear His children when they pray. Your prayers are always heard.

When I had the first set of twins, one fell ill, and the doctor's diagnosis was so scary. I went back to God and fell at His feet every minute, hour and day.
At a point, I felt like my prayers were doing nothing; I felt empty, alone, and just there. I prayed and felt nothing, heard nothing and had no dreams or prophetic encounters. Nobody called me to share what God was saying about my son, and my son grew worse. His pain and cries broke my heart into many pieces. We were constantly in and out of hospitals.

BUT! I stayed praying. I stayed there. I prayed when it felt good and when it felt empty. I prayed because I knew deep down that God could and was willing to heal him.
One day, the Lord spoke and that Word delivered my son in less than 24 hours. This was a boy who had suffered for the first five months of his life. Prayer works.

When you pray, you must BELIEVE. Faith is not how you feel; it is what you do and what you do consistently. Faith is the condition. This is the condition for answered prayers. Your faith is strengthened in Jesus' name.

Whenever you pray, and your thoughts negate your prayers, you send a mixed signal to heaven. James describes this as a double mind, saying that when we pray with a double mind, we shouldn't expect anything from God. (James 1:6-8).

When you call someone, and they put the call on hold, can you hear what they say? This is what doubt does to our prayers: it puts them on hold and hinders them from ascending to God. Have you been doubtful of whether God wants you to have children? Drive that doubt away and let this assurance settle deeply in your heart – You are a joyful mother of children. Abraham must have felt this way. Abraham hoped against hope even as he increased in age; Abraham increased more in hope and faith.

When you pray, please know that God hears and will answer you. Don't doubt this.

PRAYER

1. Thank You, Lord, for hearing me and answering my petition. Thank You for the grace to pray and pray persistently. Thank You for encouraging me and sustaining me in the place of prayer.

2. Lord, I repent from every disobedience and defiance. I am sorry for turning my back on You because I thought You turned your back on me. I felt alone, forgetting you are always there. Today, I surrender my life to you and give you complete control over my life.

3. I decree that I am strengthened to pray in Jesus' name. I pray, and I pray through in Jesus ' name. I will not be tired or weary in prayer in Jesus' name. The Right hand of God sustains me in prayer. I will break through in prayer.

4. I receive fresh fire on my prayer altar. I wake up from every spiritual slumber in Jesus' name. I come out of every discouragement, distraction and disappointment in Jesus' name. Every veil is removed in Jesus' name.

5. I receive fresh oil for prayer. The Spirit of grace and supplication rests on me afresh. (Zechariah 12:10). I will tarry in the place of prayer and abound in prayer in Jesus' name.

6. I declare that my quiver is filled with children. I am a believer, not a doubter. God hears me when I pray. When I pray, I make decrees, mountains move, crooked paths

straighten, and my life shines brighter.

7. This is the report of the Lord. I am fruitful, and I multiply. I
    am carrying my babies. God has looked upon me with favour
    and has opened my womb. I am a mother of a lovely baby
    boy, baby girl, twins, triplets, quadruplets etc. I conceive
    this year, I carry to term and deliver safely in Jesus' name.
    Amen!!! My husband will carry our babies in Jesus' name.
    Amen!

DAY 21

SUPERNATURAL FINANCIAL PROSPERITY

TEXT: Isaiah 45:3

REFLECTION:

Then you will see and be radiant, and your heart will thrill and rejoice; Because the abundance of the sea will be turned to you, the wealth of the nations will come to you. Isaiah 60:5

God wants you to prosper. He delights in the Prosperity of His children (Psalms 35:27). God wants you to have money and have lots of it. The period of waiting for a child can be expensive. You have to go for tests and procedures, and you also need to be comfortable so your mind is at rest. You cannot afford poverty or lack, and you shouldn't tolerate it.

Money amplifies. If you are going through a dark season, the lack of funds will only amplify it; this is why you should pray for financial prosperity. If you need comfort, money amplifies it. Sitting in your husband's arms in a lovely decorated room is different from being in a small and hot room where you have to break the hug to get some air. These little things might eventually lead to the big issues.

Poverty is terrible, and there is no good in it. You must hate poverty with all your heart and make no excuses for it.

Money is a defence (Ecclesiastes 7:12). There are possibilities you can access with money. God will bless the medication and procedure, but you must pay for them. Lack causes suffering to last longer and eat deeper into the soul. Poverty creates opportunities for the devil to find expression. Some arguments should not even exist, but lack will sponsor them.

When Hannah was waiting for a child, her husband gave her a double portion for the sacrifices at Shiloh. He gave her double what he gave Penniah, who had children. Why? He knows gifts can bring comfort. God's comfort is ultimate, but there are some comforts money can buy.

Lack causes strain and anger in a home. If you are constantly in disagreement, how can you host the presence of God so you can conceive supernaturally?

Prosperity helps you to live in good health conditions, feed and rest well so your body is prepared for your glorious child.

From today, you enter into much more than enough in Jesus' name.

You will lack no good thing in Jesus' name. The last time you borrowed is the last time you will ever borrow again.

Remember that God gives the power to make wealth (Deuteronomy 8:18). Honour God with your substance (Proverbs 3:9). Give your tithe, offering and help those in need. Give, and it will come back to you, good measure, pressed down, shaken together and running over (Luke 6:38).

PRAYER

1. Lord, I praise You for supplying all my needs according to Your riches in glory. (Philippians 4:19). Thank You for providing for me. Thank You for causing me to abound in all good things. (2 Corinthians 9:8).

2. Today, I declare that I have everything I need in Jesus' name. I lack no good thing, and all things are mine. God has given me all things that pertain to life and godliness. (2 Peter 1:3). Hallelujah

3. So, the (insert your family's name) became exceedingly prosperous, had large enterprises for female and male, had many servants and increased in her merchandise and estates. (Genesis 30: 43).

4. I reject every poverty mindset or attack on my life and my husband's life in Jesus' name. I cannot live in poverty or lack. I can never be stranded. God is my Shepherd, and I lack no good thing in Jesus' name. (Psalms 23:1). I reject every wind of poverty. This is not your abode in Jesus' name.

5. I call forth my supply from the four corners of the earth. Abundance flows to me from the North to the South, West and East in Jesus' name. I rise and sleep in overflowing surplus in Jesus' name.

6. My husband is a prosperous man. God has blessed the work of his hands. He is sought after and preferred above all. Our accounts are always full. We give to men just as men give to us. We are a people of God's pasture. (Psalms 100:3).

7. This is the report of the Lord. I am fruitful, and I multiply. I

am carrying my babies. God has looked upon me with favour and has opened my womb. I am a mother of a lovely baby boy, baby girl, twins, triplets, quadruplets etc. I conceive this year, I carry to term and deliver safely in Jesus' name. Amen!!! My husband will carry our babies in Jesus' name. Amen!

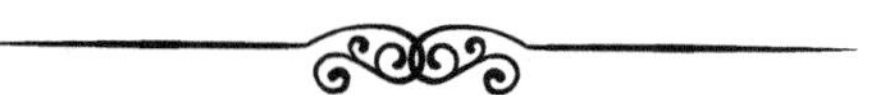

EVERY HIDDEN HEALTH PROBLEM IS EXPOSED

TEXT: LUKE 8:17

REFLECTION:

He reveals the deep and secret things: he knows what is in the darkness, and the light dwells with him. Daniel 2:22 KJV

God is light, and He wants you to live in the light, and one of the dividends of living in the light is that nothing catches you unawares. If a hidden health problem has been responsible for your inability to conceive, God wants to bring it to light so that nothing will hinder your babies from showing forth.

The enemy is heavily invested in hiding things. He can hide what is visible so you will look and not see. You must be discerning. Your discernment is increased in Jesus' name.

I know a woman who had a fibroid and could not conceive because of the fibroid. For six years, she waited. She knew she had a fibroid, but a prophet had warned her never to undergo any kind of surgery. After much prayer and encouragement, my dad encouraged her to go for surgery so the fibroid could be removed. The same year she removed the fibroid was the same year she conceived. She had her baby the following year.

The devil blinded her with fear and stopped her from correct reasoning. Your eyes are opened in Jesus' name.

I also know someone who also refused to see other doctors or go to another hospital. She used one of the best hospitals in a foreign country and did not believe anyone was more qualified than this hospital. After years of waiting, she eventually tried a local hospital in her home country after visiting many hospitals abroad. She had her baby a year after.

Ask the Lord to reveal every hidden issue and give you direction. Direction is so important. When the axe's head sank inside the river, God gave Elisha supernatural wisdom to bring it back into the open (2 Kings 6). Beyond health problems, also ask the Lord to bring everything that will benefit your overall well-being to the surface.

Lastly, keep an open mind. Believe the Lord will guide you right. Trust that He is leading you and His angels are watching over you. Pay attention to what God is saying to you and through others. Don't let your heart be fearful.

God wants to show you great and mighty things you don't know (Jeremiah 33:3). If or when He reveals anything, ask Him to guide you to the right medical professionals. Nothing remains hidden in your life anymore in Jesus' name.

PRAYER

1. Father, thank You for exposing every hidden health problem or any kind of problem in Jesus' name. Thank You for revealing the works of the enemy. Thank You for wise instructions concerning my life and my family. Thank You, Father, for light has come. (Isaiah 60:1).

2. I walk in the light, and nothing catches me unaware. Every hidden medical issue is exposed for redemption in Jesus' name. Amen. I have eyes that see and ears that hear in Jesus' name.

3. Lord, we receive direction in all we do - Who I speak with, the health facilities we use, and the doctors who work with us. Lord, let Your Holy Spirit direct us all and put the right thoughts in our hearts in Jesus' name.

4. I declare that I increase in discernment in Jesus' name. The eyes of my understanding are enlightened. I see the things hidden, and hidden things are revealed to me in Jesus' name.

5. Lord, by mercy, let the things relevant to my miracle, testimony and breakthrough be revealed to me in Jesus' name. Let mercy prevail.

6. I have found favour with God, and now all things are mine. (1 Corinthians 3:21). Every health problem is revealed and bows to the name of Jesus. I have obtained victory in Jesus' name.

7. This is the report of the Lord. I am fruitful, and I multiply. I am carrying my babies. God has looked upon me with favour and has opened my womb. I am a mother of a lovely baby boy, baby girl, twins, triplets, quadruplets etc. I conceive this year, I carry to term and deliver safely in Jesus' name. Amen!!! My husband will carry our babies in Jesus' name. Amen!

I WILL NOT MISCARRY MY BABIES

TEXT: EXODUS 23:26

REFLECTION:

Shall I bring to birth, and not cause to bring forth? Saith the Lord: shall I cause to bring forth, and shut the womb? Saith thy God.

Isaiah 66:9

God is not the author of unfinished projects. When He starts something, He completes it; He finishes what He authors and ends what He starts. God is the Alpha and Omega (Revelations 1:8). If you have been miscarrying your babies, God wants it to stop, and it stops today in Jesus' name.

Nothing makes miscarriage or stillbirth right. I know doctors have a

lot of explanations for these things, but in the beginning,
it was not so (Matthew 19:8).
The devil is the one who destroys, and he does this work by creeping into our belief system and he hides lies there so he has legal grounds to afflict us.

I had seen some friends and even family members lose their first pregnancy when I was a single lady. So, when I carried my first pregnancy and began to bleed heavily, after praying for a while, I quickly settled for a miscarriage. It was painful to accept, but my mind fell into that mould. Everything I heard from my friends and family members began to replay in my mind, and I began to say these things to myself. I believed the lie that most first-timers lose their babies because their bodies are just adjusting.

Thank God for His divine intervention through my Father in the Lord, Pastor E.A. Adeboye, who gave a word of knowledge during the May Holy Ghost Service in 2014. It was that Word that restored my faith and my fight. I eventually carried my babies to term and gave birth to two healthy babies.

Sis, you must arm yourself with God's word and stand on it. Find and listen to testimonies of those that have prevailed. We overcome by the blood of the Lamb and the Word of our testimony (Revelations 12:11). Testimonies are weapons of warfare.
Don't allow the devil to put you in any bondage of guilt and shame. If any negative feeling weighs you down, receive strength in your inner man to push it off. You will carry your babies to term and nurse them; this is God's promise for you.

Hold your womb and proclaim God's word. And stand your ground against everything that causes miscarriages and dry breasts. You will no longer cast your young and be left with an empty crib, and God will finish what He has started in you. He is Alpha and Omega.

PRAYER

1. Thank You, Lord, for You are Alpha and Omega. You are the beginning and the end. You finish what You start. You are not a man that You should lie. (Numbers 23:19).

2. I carry my babies to term and birth them alive in Jesus' name. Amen. My body is strengthened to conceive and carry to term. I rebuke every spirit of abortion in my life in Jesus' name.

3. I no longer agree with the enemy that my body cannot carry my babies to term. My body is the temple of God, and God is glorified in my body in Jesus' name. Through my pregnancy and the birth of my babies, I bring glory to God's name in Jesus' name.

4. Angels are assigned and activated to watch over me and my babies. There will be zero tolerance for satanic activities, especially against my fruitfulness in Jesus' name.

5. I will never again experience a medical error or negligence that will cost me my child. I rebuke every spirit of error in Jesus' name. I receive the grace to forgive anyone involved in the medical negligence that hurt my baby. I will not hold on to unforgiveness in Jesus' name.

6. God has given me a reason to laugh and dance for Joy. This is my season of laughter. I will laugh and dance in Jesus' name. My mourning is over.
I will dance for Joy. Hallelujah!

7. This is the report of the Lord. I am fruitful, and I multiply. I am carrying my babies. God has looked upon me with favour and has opened my womb. I am a mother of a lovely baby boy, baby girl, twins, triplets, quadruplets etc. I conceive this year, I carry to term and deliver safely in Jesus' name. Amen!!! My husband will carry our babies in Jesus' name. Amen!

DAY 24

I WILL NOT GIVE UP ON GOD

TEXT: 1 SAMUEL 30

REFLECTION:

My heart is fixed, O God, my heart is fixed: I will sing and give praise. Psalm 57:7

The devil will tempt you sore so you can give up on God. He will bring many ideas and suggestions, especially through people. He will tempt you to try other gods and ungodly methods and tempt you to seek a lover outside your marriage. He will seek to throw you in despair. You must not let him. You must resist him till he flees.

Don't give in to the devil or give up on God. 1 Timothy 6:12 says to fight a good fight of faith. You are not just fighting for your babies;

you are fighting for your faith. The enemy wants to steal your faith and take the praise of God from your life.

What will it profit a woman if she has babies but loses her soul? (Mark 8:36). Don't let the enemy break your soul. Don't give up on God.

Today's text is about David when he was faced with an impossible situation. He went on a mission and returned to find his abode burnt and his family kidnapped. His men were also faced with the same thing, and everyone wept in despair, but this was where the story took another turn.

While David's men gave up on God and wanted to stone him, David encouraged himself in the Lord and refused to give up on God. David cried, mourned his loss and then rose and encouraged himself in the Lord. It's okay to cry but don't let it break your soul. Rise from the pain and encourage yourself in the Lord.
The best time to fix your heart more firmly on God is when things are contrary. Rejoicing when things are good is normal, but rejoicing when things are contrary is supernatural.

One way to keep your heart on God and stifle the urge to give up on Him is to praise Him and remember the beautiful and wonderful things He has done in the past.

When you praise Him, your focus shifts from your problems to His power. Praise magnifies the power of God and reveals His limitless abilities. Do you feel like throwing in the towel? Throw up your praise instead. Get your musical instruments. You can use your pots and frying pan if you don't have any, and give God some quality praise today. You will find new strength and grace as you release your praise to heaven. Dance your way into your miracle.

PRAYER

1. Thank you, Jesus, the owner of my soul. Alpha and Omega, You are worthy to be praised. In all generations, there is no one like You. You are the only one worthy to be praised.

2. Lord, You know my deepest thoughts. I am sorry for all the sinful thoughts I allowed because I was tempted to give up. I repent from them all and surrender my life to You completely.

3. Father, please hold me by the hand. Give me fresh reassurance. Don't let me fail You in this great test. Don't let me give up on You. I have no power of my own.

4. I ask for strength, Lord, strengthen me. Let your strength overtake me. Lord Jesus, touch my weary heart and let it come alive with Your strength in Jesus' name.

5. In the name of Jesus, I break the stronghold of discouraging and lustful thoughts in my mind in Jesus' name. I close off every access point of the enemy into my mind in Jesus' name. I pull down every imagination against God in my heart in Jesus' name.

6. Today, I lie beside the still waters, and the Lord, the Shepherd of my soul, restores me in Jesus' name. I am completely restored. I am back on my feet and will not give up on God in Jesus' name.

7. This is the report of the Lord. I am fruitful, and I multiply. I am carrying my babies. God has looked upon me with favour and has opened my womb. I am a mother of a lovely baby boy, baby girl, twins, triplets, quadruplets etc. I conceive this year, I carry to term and deliver safely in Jesus' name. Amen!!! My husband will carry our babies in Jesus' name. Amen!

LORD, SEND ME ENCOURAGERS

TEXT: 1 CHRONICLES 12:22

REFLECTION:

I will not leave you comfortless: I will come to you. John 14:18
KJV

Encouragement is a soul tonic that makes the heart strong. Everyone needs encouragement, and it is your responsibility to ask for it when needed. Don't wait for people to encourage you. Encourage yourself and ask your close allies to encourage you when you feel down. Sometimes, people don't know what we need because we look all put together.

When was the last time you asked someone to pray for you, hug you, or send you a word of encouragement?

Ask, and you shall receive (Matthew 7:7). Today is a good day to ask for encouragement.

When Jesus was about to leave, He gave His disciples the promise of the Holy Spirit. He promised them that He would not leave them without comfort and encouragement. This word is for you also. Jesus will not leave you without encouragement and encouragers; He will come to you.

In our text, God sent men daily to David to strengthen his hands until the kingdom was given to him. God's declaration in the beginning that it is not good for man to be alone still stands, and He will not leave you to stand alone in this season. (Genesis 2:18).

God can encourage you through anything: songs, books, nature, circumstances, anything! He can even encourage you through the people who have discouraged you.

You must also learn to be to others what you want them to be to you. Encourage people greatly. Encourage them with your substance, presence, time, skills, words, attitude etc.

You will not be without helpers and encouragers in this season, beloved sister. God will come to you.

PRAYER

1. Thank You, Lord, for the oil of gladness. Thank You, for You have rolled away the darkness in my soul and given me joy. Thank You for encouraging me greatly. I am grateful that You have revived my soul.

2. I do not lack encouragement in this season. God sends encouragement as and when I need it in Jesus' name. Amen. I am fortified on all sides by the sound of encouragement.

3. I silence the voice of discouragement in Jesus' name. I come out of every association sponsoring fear and discouragement in my life in Jesus' name.

4. I find favour with my loved ones in Jesus' name. They carry me in their heart and do not despise me in Jesus' name. God has spotlighted me before my spouse, pastors, mentors, parents and loved ones so I can find the encouragement I need this season.

5. I break free from hopelessness and fear. I will not be a captive of fear and discouragement in Jesus' name. I am free from every thought of depression in Jesus' name.

6. Today, I draw strength from God and encourage myself in the Lord. I rise from ashes to beauty, mourning to dancing and trade the spirit of heaviness for a garment of praise in Jesus' name.

7. This is the report of the Lord. I am fruitful, and I multiply. I am carrying my babies. God has looked upon

me with favour and has opened my womb. I am a mother of a lovely baby boy, baby girl, twins, triplets, quadruplets etc. I conceive this year, I carry to term and deliver safely in Jesus' name. Amen!!! My husband will carry our babies in Jesus' name. Amen!

LORD, DEFEND ME FROM THOSE THAT MOCK ME

TEXT: PSALM 3

REFLECTION:

As birds flying, so will the Lord of hosts defend Jerusalem (Put your name); defending also, he will deliver it; and passing over, he will preserve it. Isaiah 31:5

Mockery, like praise, is a powerful weapon. Don't underestimate the effect of mockery. Mockery can turn a king into a coward. Mockery can break a soul and render it hopeless.

The purpose of mockery is to provoke sorrow and anger. Those who mock you do so to make you sad and angry; don't let them. Use their mockery as an avenue to receive the strength to pray.

The Bible says a mocker is a fool (Psalms 74:22), wicked (Psalms 1:1) and hater of knowledge (Proverbs 1:22). These people are also enemies of God (Psalms 74:10). God has promised that anyone who sows mockery will reap the same (Galatians 6:7).

Nehemiah took up a noble task, yet he was mocked by haters of God. Despite the mockery, Nehemiah refused to be deterred. He persisted and continued to make progress until he eventually finished the work (Nehemiah 4). Don't let your Mockers stop you from doing what God put in your heart. Don't let their mockery stop you from believing and declaring your faith in God.

As Peninnah mocked Hannah, you might also have people who taunt, belittle or say hurtful words to your face. (1 Samuel 1:6). Don't harbour hatred towards them for their words and actions. Let God fight for you.

When Sennacherib sent a letter to Hezekiah mocking his faith in God, Hezekiah took that letter to the temple and laid it before God. God's response to that act of surrender was sending an angel who killed one hundred and eighty-five thousand soldiers in the enemy's camp (2 Kings 18 and 19). If that is not God's defence, I don't know what is!

God doesn't defend those whose words are sharp, wise and strong enough to defend themselves. He defends those who put their trust in Him. God's way of defending Hannah from Peninnah's mockery wasn't to kill Peninnah or inflict her with sickness; His defence was to give Hannah proof – Samuel and the other children. God gave Hannah a star child - a child who led an entire nation for years.

Today, ask the Lord to defend you by giving you proof and watch Him do beyond your greatest expectations.

PRAYER

1. Thank You, Lord, for defending me against my mockers and scorners. Thank You for fighting for me. Thank You, for my soul will not be sorrowful or vexed by what people say against me. I know my time has come, and everyone will rejoice with me in Jesus' name.

2. I declare that the Lord hears me on the day of trouble; the name of the God of Jacob defends me. He sends me help from His sanctuary. Amen. (Psalm 20:1-2). I am not without help.

3. As the Lord gave Hannah a glorious child, I receive my glorious children too. My womb will carry my children this year, and I will deliver them safely in Jesus' name.

4. I declare that my heart will not be bitter or broken. I rise above the evil words of men. I will not be afraid of their voices or faces. I will love and pray for them no matter what they do. I choose love.

5. God has made me a name and a praise. Reproach and mockery are not my portion. It comes to an end now. I decree an end to every mockery in Jesus' name. (Zephaniah 3:19).

6. I frustrate every voice mocking me and every agenda to make me a subject of mockery. It will not stand in Jesus' name. People who have decided to mock me will be victims of their plans in Jesus' name. Every mocker of

my life will be disgraced and put to shame in Jesus' name.

7.   This is the report of the Lord. I am fruitful, and I multiply. I am carrying my babies. God has looked upon me with favour and has opened my womb. I am a mother of a lovely baby boy, baby girl, twins, triplets, quadruplets etc. I conceive this year, I carry to term and deliver safely in Jesus' name. Amen!!! My husband will carry our babies in Jesus' name. Amen!

MY HUSBAND'S HEART WILL NOT BE WEARY

TEXT: MATTHEW 11:28-30

REFLECTION:

He gives strength to the weary and increases the power of the weak. Isaiah 40:29

Often, more attention and help are directed at women trusting God for a child because of the assumption that men are strong. Men are strong, but they are human. They have feelings, and as the head of the home, the waiting period can be a heavy weight to bear. Some men have suffered depression because of this. No matter how strong a man is, he needs prayers and affection.

Hannah's husband must have felt the weight of waiting for a child. In a bid to make his wife happy, he asked in desperation if he wasn't worth more than ten sons to her (1 Samuel 1:8). He sounded like a tired man who didn't know what to do.

Your husband needs all the prayer and encouragement he can get. It is not easy for a man to wait for a child he can call his own. It is not easy for him to watch you ache for something he cannot give you. Your pain multiplies his pain. He may even feel defeated. He may not say or show it because he needs to be strong for you, but you can rest assured that he thinks about it a lot.

Please, encourage your husband or any man waiting on God for a child to speak out. Encourage them to go for therapy, or take a break from work and even from home to go somewhere they can relax and reconnect with God deeply.

One of the devil's tactics to pull down people is to send the spirit of discouragement against them. He did this to Elijah after he (Elijah) confronted Baal and his worshippers in Israel. (1 Kings 19). Discouragement makes the heart heavy and weary, making people unable to pray and seek God fervently. Another effect of discouragement is that it sows the seed of doubt and unbelief in God's promises and makes people quit their assignments.

As your home's gatekeeper, don't let discouragement weigh your husband's heart down. When you sense its operations, fight against it in prayers. You can also ask the Lord to open your eyes so you can sense it and fortify your borders before it strikes.

When you see your husband tired of the wait, strengthen his heart in prayers. Speak life over him and to him. Hug him. Be the voice of hope. Both of you should strengthen each other. Like Aaron and Hur strengthened the hands of Moses until Israel conquered the Amalekites, hold your husband up until he becomes strong again to keep holding on (Exodus 17).

When a man loses hope, the home falls apart. Pray for your husband; don't let your home fall apart.

Couples waiting for the fruit of the womb must be gentle and patient with each other.

PRAYER

1. Father, thank You for my husband. Thank You for keeping him in good health and sound mind. Thank You for how far You have brought my husband. Thank You for not letting the enemy break his soul.

2. I speak life over my husband. You (call his name) will not be weary, discouraged or tired. You will not give up on God. Your future is great and blessed in Jesus' name. Together, we will see the fulfilment of God's promises over us. Amen.

3. (Insert your husband's name), I speak peace over your mind in Jesus' name. Your mind is shielded from every negative thought in Jesus' name. Your mind will not be troubled in Jesus' name.

4. You will not give up on God in Jesus' name. You rise above every despair and shame in Jesus' name. You will not lose your patience with God.

5. Daily, you increase in strength. God will comfort you when you feel low and weary. Your strength is renewed, and your hope is strengthened in Jesus' name. Your eyes see clearly in Jesus' name.

6. I ask the Lord to surround you with safe and godly association that will strengthen and encourage you in Jesus' name. God orders your steps into the right relationships in Jesus' name. You are surrounded by godly fathers, mentors

and good friends in Jesus' name.

7. This is the report of the Lord. I am fruitful, and I multiply. I am carrying my babies. God has looked upon me with favour and has opened my womb. I am a mother of a lovely baby boy, baby girl, twins, triplets, quadruplets etc. I conceive this year, I carry to term and deliver safely in Jesus' name. Amen!!! My husband will carry our babies in Jesus' name. Amen!

A STRANGE WOMAN WILL NOT COME INTO MY HOME

TEXT: 2 SAMUEL 22:46

REFLECTION:

For we are not fighting against human beings but against the wicked spiritual forces in the heavenly world, the ruler, authorities, and cosmic powers of this dark age. Ephesians 6:12 GNT

The devil does not play fair! He plays dirty, and he plays bad. He wants to take advantage of you and your spouse at this time. He wants to corrupt your lineage and legacy. He wants to plant seeds of discord and steal your peace. He wants to bring Jezebel into your home.

Adultery is not the way to have a child. Sin is never the way. It may make sense, but it is not of God and will cost you your soul. The blessing of God adds no sorrow (Proverbs 10:22).

Don't encourage your husband to seek another woman for the sake of having a child, nor should you seek a lover who can give you a child. Don't take from the devil what God can give you.

Sarah invited trouble into her home when she asked her husband to take Hagar as a concubine so she could have a child through her. She didn't know she had invited someone that would contend with God's promises for her home, child and future generations. Strange people often don't start out as strange; they might look innocent and harmless, but their presence will eventually do more harm than good in the long run.

A strange woman doesn't necessarily have to be another woman who wants to ruin your home; she can be anything that wants to contend with God's promises concerning your children. Strange friends, ideas and philosophies also fall into this category, and you must learn to discern what you allow into your space.

Don't fall into the trap Sarah fell into, and try to use others to bring God's promises to pass in your life because it will backfire and become a thorn in your flesh later. And if another woman is already positioning herself to win your husband's heart, root her out in the place of prayers. If another man has become your heart's desire, you must confess it to the Lord and cut off any communication with the man.

It is common practice for many people trying to conceive to try out with others, but this practice is very demonic. Fornication and adultery are demonic. Don't invite the devil into your home. The spiritual, mental, emotional and financial damage is often generational.

There are strangers waiting for the right time to jump into your home. May the Lord protect you from them in Jesus' name.

Ask the Lord to fish every stranger out of their hidden places and to reveal those things, people and ideas that will oppose His will in your life now and in the future.

PRAYER

1. Thank You, Lord, for Your hedge around my home. Thank You, Father, for disconnecting me and my partner from anyone who wants to bring a stranger into our home.

2. Father, please help my husband and I to stay strong and overcome every temptation in Jesus' name. We do not break our vow before you and men in Jesus' name.

3. I declare that I don't allow strangers into my heart and marriage knowingly and unknowingly. And every stranger in my home or around me becomes uncomfortable and flees out of their hiding place in Jesus' name.

4. Lord, any woman or man who has decided to come between my husband and I, let your fire fall on them in Jesus' name. Anyone waiting for the perfect moment to defile my matrimonial bed is uprooted from our lives in Jesus' name.

5. Lord, separate my husband and I from anyone influencing and seducing us to consider strange husbands or wives in Jesus' name. My marriage will not be disgraced or destroyed. My marriage is fortified and preserved by God. God is invested in my home, and anyone who seeks its downfall will see the wrath of God.

6. We will not fail you, Lord. We will stand strong and pure in Jesus' name like the three Hebrew boys. Our lives will glorify you in Jesus' name.

7. This is the report of the Lord. I am fruitful, and I multiply.
    I am carrying my babies. God has looked upon me with
    favour and has opened my womb. I am a mother of a
    lovely baby boy, baby girl, twins, triplets, quadruplets etc.
    I conceive this year, I carry to term and deliver safely in
    Jesus' name. Amen!!! My husband will carry our babies in
    Jesus' name. Amen!

MY MARRIAGE WILL STAND STRONG

TEXT: PSALM 112

REFLECTION:

Those who trust in the Lord are as unshakeable, as immovable as mighty Mount Zion. Psalm 125: 1 TPT

I know this is a tough season for you and your spouse. Every marriage goes through trying seasons but delay in childbearing hits differently. This is not the time to think you made a wrong choice, nor the time to think your partner's past is haunting you. Instead, let James 1:2-4 be your testimony. Let this trial strengthen your faith and perfect your character. Allow this to make your marriage better.

The waiting period can either strengthen or break a marriage. Many homes have cracked under the weight of waiting, but yours doesn't have to. This is a season to get more knowledge and transform your knowledge into wisdom because knowledge and wisdom will be the stability of your times. (Isaiah 33:6).

As you seek wisdom, get understanding too. Seek to understand your spouse more and never take him for granted. Please don't give him the impression that he is the reason you are yet to conceive. Allow your love for him to fill every part of your heart.
Don't just wait for things to happen; Get involved in Kingdom business and pour yourself into diligent service. You can also have some children from your siblings or close family friends sleep over at your house from time to time. You can experience the joy of children from time to time through other children. You can learn a new skill with your spouse, go on missionary trips and visit new places worldwide.

Delay is not a death sentence. It is an extension of a season in your life. You can either enjoy your waiting or make your life miserable. Choose to enjoy your waiting.

Also, read books on parenting and prepare yourself actively for the coming of your children. Wisdom will make your home strong, and understanding will establish it. While you pray that the Lord will fortify your home from evil external influences, your wisdom will seal every crack in the wall that can allow them to slither in.

Give attention to the Word of God and prayer. Guard your home with intense prayers. Be gentle with each other. Keep your intimacy warm and cosy. Enjoy each other. Prioritize the bond you share because you will be left with each other long after your children start their lives.

When you apply wisdom and seek knowledge and understanding, your home will withstand the storms that tear other homes apart.

God will make your home a shining star in Jesus' name.

PRAYER

1. Thank You for keeping my home in perfect peace and joy. Thank You, Lord.

2. Lord, you have commanded that we love each other. We receive fresh love and affection for each other in Jesus' name. Our love for each other will not be frustrated in Jesus' name. Lord, increase Your love in our hearts in Jesus' name.

3. Lord, let Your kingdom and dominion reign in my marriage in Jesus' name. Let no contrary spirit or voice find expression in my home in Jesus' name.

4. I decree that my are of one spirit and mind in Jesus' name. We are bound in heart and mind. Our language is one; we are not divided in Jesus' name.

5. Father, help us to identify the work You are doing for us. Lord, help us to please You so we can continually reach higher levels of unity in our marriage – spiritually, physically, and mentally.

6. I am wise; therefore, I am strong, and my home is strong. I am a woman of knowledge, and I increase in strength. The storms that destroy other homes will only make my home stronger and better in Jesus' name. Amen.

7. This is the report of the Lord. I am fruitful, and I multiply. I am carrying my babies. God has looked upon me with favour and has opened my womb. I am a mother of a

lovely baby boy, baby girl, twins, triplets, quadruplets etc.
I conceive this year, I carry to term and deliver safely in
Jesus' name. Amen!!! My husband will carry our babies in
Jesus' name. Amen!

I WILL NOT GIVE UP HOPE

TEXT: ROMANS 4:16-22

REFLECTION:

Now the God of hope fill you with all joy and peace in believing that you may abound in hope, through the power of the Holy Ghost. Romans 15:13 KJV

Look at how far you have come, sis. Look at all God has done for you. I know this is hard, but you cannot afford to give up hope. You are no ordinary person; you are a BELIEVER. Believing is what we do because God is real. To lose hope is to say God cannot do this.

I charge you to stand firm, stand like a warrior, stand like a Son and stand victorious.

Hope is no wishful thinking. It is premised on the assured promises of God. The Word of God is incapable of failing.

Hope is a supernatural strategy for every believer. As long as there is hope, there will be life, and hope fuels faith because faith is the substance of things hoped for (Hebrews 11:1). God wants to fill your heart with hope so that your hope can strengthen you to keep believing against all odds as Abraham did.

If there is anyone that should give up hope in the Scriptures, Abraham and Sarah are more than qualified. Yet, the Scripture records that Abraham didn't look at his dead body or Sarah's womb. Despite his hopeless circumstances, he kept his hope alive. He believed he would father nations despite the contrary report his body and the world told him. You also must keep your hope alive. Go where there is hope, listen to messages that revive your hope, surround yourself with people of hope, listen to the testimonies of others and break away from naysayers.

Regardless of the report you have heard or what you see daily, choose to hope against hope.

Tell yourself this, *'I WILL NOT GIVE UP HOPE.'* Habakkuk 3:17-19.

Once Satan can puncture your hope, he can harvest your reality. Don't allow him! When God gives you hope, the results are joy, peace and more hope and never forget that hope never disappoints.

God will always come through for those whose hopes are alive.

Your breakthrough is here. The child you prayed for is here. Don't lose hope. You, too, will be a mother of many children. This is the report of the Lord; believe it.

PRAYER

1. Habakkuk 3:19 (KJV) Thank You, Lord, for You are my strength, and You have made my feet like hinds' feet, and You have made me walk upon mine high places. Thank You, Jesus.

2. Father, renew the hope of my marriage. I decree in the name of Jesus that my marriage will not be hopeless. My marriage rises above every storm and challenge in Jesus' name.

3. Every good thing my marriage needs to prosper is supplied in Jesus' name. Good things come to me and my husband in Jesus' name. We are filled with God's goodness in Jesus' name.

4. My marriage is filled with joy and laughter in Jesus' name. Only shouts of joy are heard in my home. Those waiting for the downfall of my home will be ashamed in Jesus' name.

5. This time next year, by the mercy of God, my will carry our babies in our arms. People will rejoice with us in Jesus' name.

6. Lord, you are the shield, glory and lifter of my marriage. While we wait for the miracle of a child, I ask that You fill my marriage with Your manifold glory in Jesus' name.

7. This is the report of the Lord. I am fruitful, and I multiply. I am carrying my babies. God has looked upon me with favour and has opened my womb. I am a mother of a lovely

baby boy, baby girl, twins, triplets, quadruplets etc.
I conceive this year, I carry to term and deliver safely in
Jesus' name. Amen!!! My husband will carry our babies in
Jesus' name. Amen!

LORD JESUS, CARRY ME THROUGH

TEXT: ISAIAH 41:13

REFLECTION:

Listen to me, family of Jacob (Put your family's name), everyone that's left of the family of Israel, I've been carrying you on my back from the day you were born, And I'll keep carrying you when you are old. I'll be there, bearing you up when you are old and gray. I've done it and will keep on doing it, carrying you on my back, saving you. Isaiah 46:3-4 MSG

Congratulations, Mother of Nations. I congratulate you because nations are inside you, waiting to be born.

You have journeyed through these 31 days with great anticipation and hope, and your hope is becoming a reality.

This new phase of birthing your promises will stretch you, but you have nothing to worry about because you have been prepared for such a time as this (Esther 4:14). As you move from waiting to birthing, open your arms and ask the Lord to carry you. God loves to do you good and wants to make you a showpiece of His glory and beauty. He wants to beautify you with all the dividends of salvation, one of which is the gift of children.

He is faithful to complete what He has started and will surpass your expectations. In this transition period, draw closer to God than ever before. When the devil cannot stop a baby from being conceived, he always fights to stop its birth. Ask the Lord to carry you; He will bear you through eagle's wings. God's grace is enough to carry you through all the phases ahead. Expect Him to show up for you every time.

I encourage you to listen to Minister Nathaniel Bassey's song 'Holy Spirit, carry me'. Allow God to carry you in this phase and all the days of your life. It will bring you great rest and replenish your soul.

God loves the vulnerable, and He loves to be our Superman. Depend totally on Him and watch Him carry you to greater heights of Glory.

Congratulations once again, sis.

PRAYER

1. Thank you, Lord, for Your faithfulness to me and my husband. You have carried me all these years. You have been my help, my defence and my glory.

2. The Lord carries me through this season and every season ahead. He bears me up on eagle's wings, and I will not be weary. God will keep my feet steady, and He will plant my feet on solid ground.

3. I go from strength to strength, glory to glory and victory to victory. The Lord is my strength, and I will not fall. My heart is strengthened in Jesus' name.

4. *He tends his flock like a shepherd: He gathers the lambs in his arms and carries them close to his heart; He gently leads those that have young. Isaiah 40:11.* Lord, carry me close to Your heart. Let me know, and feel Your reassuring presence.

5. As You carry me, Lord, shift my gaze to You. Let me see the wonders of Your presence, glory and power. Let my eyes see as You see, and my ears hear as You hear.

6. Lord, carry me and my babies to term and safe delivery. Carry everyone that will participate in the delivery of my children so their hands work as Yours. There will be no error or mistake in Jesus' name.

7. This is the report of the Lord. I am fruitful, and I multiply. I am carrying my babies. God has looked upon me with

favour and has opened my womb. I am a mother of a lovely baby boy, baby girl, twins, triplets, quadruplets etc. I conceive this year, I carry to term and deliver safely in Jesus' name. Amen!!! My husband will carry our babies in Jesus' name. Amen!

TESTIMONIES

"Mine was a different case. I have had 2 children before and was trusting God for a male child.When I was ready conception wasn't happening. So I joined the supernatural child birth group through the warrior mom's prayer hub. We had prayer partners and we faithfully carried out the prayer sessions as instructed. There were also reviews of testimonies from people who had waited for years and how God came through for them. After a month that I joined, the Lord came through. I had another Baby Girl which was the Lord's best gift for me like he revealed to me when I was about 7 months pregnant or there about. Not a boy as I so desired but 2 years plus now, the traits and everything about her has proved that she is indeed the best of God for me."
-Oluyomi Ibukun.

"Good evening ma. I have come to give God all the glory. Barely a month after the "rain of babies" program held in September 2022. After my myectomy in 2021 my doctor told me my 2 fallopian tubes were blocked and I couldn't conceive except through IVF. To God be the glory. I have conceived naturally without any form of aid. God has shown me mercy. Please praise the Lord for me.

What the doctors called impossible, God has done it."
-Victoria

"Heaven smiled on us and blessed us with a Daughter! After waiting 9 years. 5 failed IVf! 9 failed IUI! Still birth at 42 weeks! Years of sorry and agony came to an end. Family celebrate with me am finally a MUM."
-Olubunmi Ibidunni

"Thank God for the amazing 31 days. I remember the day you told those trusting God to write down their EDD. By faith, I did this and kept praying. Sis, in less than how many days the lord has done it o. I did a home test on the 1st of Dec and it came back positive. I just kept shouting "Irorun lo ba de" that was another word that came forth from the prayer challenge. God is so good....baby No.2 is on the way. Hallelujah.
God bless you abundantly sis. Good Morning. God has done it again! He not only answered the prayer of conception, he saw me through the entire journey and granted a safe delivery. Baby No.2 is here to the glory of God. Wanted to share with the sent mothers because the prayer was raised on November 2021's prayer challenge."
-Anonymous

"Good morning ma, I want to testify to the Glory of God, his love Fatherly is immeasurable, indeed I have seen the Lord's goodness and mercy. I am the one God has shown Mercy. Last year was my most dark moments and everything seems grumbling before my face till I became depressed and suicidal, I tried to seek God but

he seems so far... I entered this year struggling, my marriage was crashing, my vision for life was blur I couldn't see a way out, till I encountered SENT MOTHERS IN MARCH, BY the HOLY SPIRIT HIMSELF ... I DON'T WATCH SPONSORED AD ON FACEBOOK BUT SOMEHOW I WATCH THAT OF THE FESTIVAL OF FIRE, I felt I should attended which was on my wedding anniversary day, I registered for both online and onsite but couldn't attend any because that day, the devil came for my home... Subsequently I started listening to the Mondays and Thursdays prayers... And my relationship with God was built. Before I skipped what Happened March 17 we discovered I was pregnant. I was falling ill severally after treatment of Malaria and infection and then decided to go for a test. Then we discovered on our 5th year anniversary day that I was pregnant. Last year I also felt a certain way that we were only taking care of children without following the program but I didn't know we were the first partakers. I have been trusting God for a baby for 2years and i found out I was pregnant immediately I came back from the blossom convention and I had my baby on the 24th of December 2022. That was the reason I couldn't attend physically this year I could only join online. Children teachers are indeed the first partakers!!!"
-Anonymous

"I had secondary Infertility. In my waiting period, my emotions was all over the place, going for naming ceremonies of friends and younger cousins got me feeling less of myself. I am grateful for my husband, he stood grounds for me at the family front especially his, at some point he ordered his dad not to ask or call me mama Ibeji, as time went by my FIL became the one standing his grounds for me

but he still kept the mama Ibeji name (haha).

Medically there was fibroids, I had a myomectomy in an hospital in Lagos, it was a very trying time for me as post op my body was not absorbing the stitches and it was popping out of the stitch line on my tummy, we went back and they had to pull the thread off me(the pain I will not forget in a hurry) but afterwards I healed and was ready but baby didn't come, I was told to do hydrotubation to flush my fallopian tubes lo and behold no baby yet, we had spent so much money but God raised helpers for our sake, we decided to go for IVF so all the pre tests before the procedure showed that I had bilateral hydrosalpinx (means water in both my fallopian tubes) and the fertility doctor at that time advised my husband and I to clip both my tubes so that the water from the tubes won't affect when the embryo is transferred, we decided to in 2019 but right before the procedure started I mean I was already on the surgery table. Drips and injections already in my veins and all of a sudden, I started gasping for breath and coughing I asked the nurse the name of the injection she just gave me and she said it's paracetamol but I kept gasping and the Doctor came in and said he was sorry we cannot continue the procedure as they do not he the facility for an emergency and my body is not ready for the procedure, I got back to my husband in the waiting room and he simply said I know God will give us our children let's go home.

I still did the IVF months later and it failed, I immediately went to Instagram and used the #ivf #infertility and I was simply opened another account @fertilerae and got more information but we weren't buoyant enough for a second round immediately so I kept posting prophetically and praying to testify someday soon, the

IVF failed February 2020 and I just decided to stop stressing and stopped all the drugs and simply led a healthy lifestyle and eating habit. By my birthday (September) in 2020 I was sad my red robots came again and I decided not to celebrate, the Holy Spirit called my attention to the fact that I am still alive and I still have hope, I chose to be happy again, I celebrated my birthday and by October 2020 I found out that I was pregnant, I was on my second dose of Lonart when my husband begged me to stop, felt like I was the last person to get in terms with me being pregnant! To the Glory of God I welcomed by Princess in June of 2021!

Trust me I had a great relief because my husband kept praying and I simply took to singing praises I listened to worship music, I have a playlist from Ebe by Sola Allyson to Gratitude by Tope Alabi and at some point we were fasting and praying too, when I feel weak in my spirit I just listen to worship songs and crying to God for my miracle.

I want to thank God for the group created for waiting mothers by Sent Mothers Global Prayer Hub, it strengthened me most especially the declarations, there was a particular declaration we had sometimes in 2020 I didn't even know I was already pregnant. I joined the SUPERNATURAL FRUITFULNESS CIRCLE through by best friend (Jumoke) she saw the link and sent it to me, I was skeptical at first so she joined in with me too; she did that to support me. The group really strengthened me especially the declarations, the 2020 declaration. I also remember a time we were also asked to call fellow sisters on the group and pray together mine were sisters Damilola and Busayo. A big shout out to you too!

I also listened to moms in the Supernatural Fruitfulness Circle